Thin From Within

The Proven Breakthrough to Take It Off and Keep It Off

By Steve Webster C.Ht

Thin From Within

The Proven Breakthrough to Take It Off and Keep It Off

By Steve Webster C.Ht

Edited by Melanie M. Morgan

CONTENTS

Chapter 1: Why Am I Overweight?

You may have tried dieting all your life. Sometimes experiencing periods of success, only to see the weight return, and then some. Dieting alone does not work. Especially long term. If it did, you wouldn't be reading this book.

No matter how strong your desire to be thin, to be your perfect weight, to be healthy, you've fallen short. You may blame yourself, your metabolism, your spouse for tempting you with fattening foods, your kids for leaving their mac-n-cheese half eaten. You may have even raised the white flag and given up. And who would blame you? There are millions of others like you, in the very same spot - frustrated, tired, and disheartened. Having tried everything and finding that nothing seems to work. That is, until now.

When you have approached weight loss in the past, it was likely with a diet, and perhaps exercise. And sure, those are key ingredients you would expect to work. But what they lacked was the most powerful weapon in your weight loss arsenal: ***your mind.***

This book will explain why your mind is the primary reason you are overweight, and how to harness the power of your subconscious mind, which will make weight loss a definite, gradual, inevitable, unstoppable process.

Dieting is no fun, and the results are generally short term. Is there a way to lose the excess weight permanently? The short answer is: absolutely! Most of us have tried to diet at one point or another. And perhaps we were successful TEMPORARILY – we lost 2 pounds, 5 pounds or even 10 pounds. But it was not very long before our old friend (adipose tissue) returned, especially to the problem areas on our body.

Diets are a temporary solution and have no long-term guarantees. In fact, quite the opposite is true, as you will learn later in this book. Only rarely does the weight stay off permanently from dieting alone.

Diets also evoke feelings of deprivation and pain. To me, the word DIET stands for:

- **D**elicious **I**ngredients **E**liminated **T**oday
- **D**isappointed **I**t **E**nhanced **T**emporarily
- **D**oesn't **I**mprove **E**verlasting **T**ransformation
- **D**id **I** **E**at Today?

Permanent weight loss is achieved through making lifestyle changes. These lifestyle changes can be embraced and driven by your core program which resides in your subconscious. You, your body image, and your body size, have manifested from who you are, your lifestyle, and how you have been programmed since birth.

You can rewrite that subconscious program, so that you embrace lifestyle changes willingly, and without a feeling of deprivation. If you do not rewrite this program, then every time you lose weight, your subconscious will trigger actions to revert to what is called 'homeostasis', (which

means to stay the same; at its 'norm'; or a 'set-point').
The subconscious does not like 'unknowns'. No matter
how desirable the unknown may be (such as a newly trim
body), it is unfamiliar and perceived as a threat by the
subconscious mind. We can change this programming so
that your perfect weight becomes your new level of
homeostasis: the image the subconscious has of what you
look like, and how much you weigh.

With so many people desperate to lose weight, spending
time, effort and money, only to achieve limited gains, the
only people winning are the people selling the latest fad
diets, fad nutrients, or fad medications.

But weight loss **can** be easy, automatic and permanent if
you only change one thing – **your mind**! When you
previously attempted a diet, you did it with your
conscious mind – only. But your conscious mind is only
10% of your mind's power. Your **subconscious** mind is
90%, which makes it many times more powerful. When
you engage your subconscious mind, along with your
conscious mind, you are applying 100% to your diet goals
(or any goal for that matter) and they will no longer
sabotage one another, which has been the reason for
your weight loss frustrations.

Using hypnosis alone, I lost 14 pounds in 1 month – and it
was easy! Every month I continue to lose weight, gain
muscle and become healthier – doing nothing more than
the process I outline in this book. The best thing is that
these changes are permanent. I never have to worry
about being overweight again.

If you are overweight, it is likely due to multiple causes. And these causes can be a complicated process of factors that can be summed with the acronym F.A.T.N.E.S.S., as well as a not-so-catchy acronym H.I.M.G.

'FATNESS' contains the primary causes of the body moving from its natural lean state to an overweight state:

- **F**ood Addiction/Over-Eating
- **A**lcohol
- **T**oxins
- **N**arcotics/Meds
- **E**motions
- **S**tress
- **S**leep

These are the primary catalysts for weight gain, which lead to the secondary causes. Inflammation is a contributor to being overweight, but inflammation occurs as a direct result of what we eat, drink, the toxins we consume or are exposed to, stress and lack of sleep. Similarly, your gut biome is incredibly important in determining whether you are lean or obese, and this too is primarily a result of what we ingest.

Hormones are another major factor, but again, hormones are dependent on the items listed and are a side-effect of several of them. One might argue: 'but I have thyroid issues which lead to a hormone imbalance.' If a person were to eat properly, reduce alcohol and stimulants, remove toxins, avoid unnecessary medications, achieve emotional balance, relax more, stress less and experience quality sleep, then this would eliminate the clear majority of illness (including the thyroid) and behavioral disorders. Finally, your metabolism is the primary indicator of whether you are lean or overweight. We all know people who can eat whatever they want, and as much as they want, and yet remain slim. Similarly, we all know people who hardly eat anything at all and cannot become lean. The reason is our metabolic rate, the rate at which our bodies burn up the fuel we put into them. When you limit your calorie intake, the subconscious mind acknowledges the reduced amount of fuel and slows down your metabolic rate accordingly. This is a basic survival mechanism. For all it knows, you are in the mountains next to a crashed airplane, trying to stay alive. So even if your metabolism started off pretty good, you, in essence, shut it down by dieting. Then due to that same survival instinct, it holds onto whatever it can get when you finally do eat, which ends up stored as fat later.

Our acronym FATNESS works hand in hand with the secondary issues, Hormones, Inflammation, Gut-Biome, and Metabolism (HIMG). As you can see, weight management is a complicated process of balancing multiple factors. It is not as simple as just reducing calories or 30 minutes on the treadmill for instance.

So now we are aware of why we continue to battle with weight issues, no matter how hard we work at them. How do we rectify this? We begin with another acronym I call 'PRIMER':

- **P**hysical Exercise
- **R**educe Stress
- Increase Metabolism
- **M**ental & Physical Detox
- **E**ngage the Subconscious
- **R**ectify Nutrition

Most diets focus only on calorie intake, which is a minor element. And no diets focus on the most important aspect: *your mind.*

This book will teach you a permanent 'solution' to the weight issues you've been fighting, as well as how to enjoy continued weight management...*for life!* The best part about it all is that you can do it YOURSELF. You don't need to spend thousands of dollars going to 'experts' who only help you achieve short term gains, if any at all.

In this book, we will discuss how the mind is responsible for weight gain (and therefore weight loss), the importance of your metabolism and your gut biome, and the importance of nutrition in your healthy lifestyle.

Each of these aspects is important on its own; but when combined, they work synergistically to help you achieve more weight loss, in a shorter period, and with a more permanent result. The whole is infinitely more powerful than the sum of the parts. But by far the most important aspect of whether you are lean or overweight is your mind (i.e., your mindset and your subconscious programming).

We are all aware of the many benefits associated with weight loss:

- Self-Confidence
- Attractiveness/Desirability
- Inner Resolve
- Health
- Well-Being
- Self-Esteem
- Role Model (for kids or significant other)
- Clothes Fit Better
- Exercise Becomes Easier
- Sports/Athletic Efficiency
- Increased Energy
- Improved Emotional State

Of course, a lean and healthy body is highly desirable. Why then have you not achieved this lofty goal? There are many reasons. The most impactful is this: you have consciously decided that you want to lose weight; BUT your inner programming of who you are, and how you behave, reside in your subconscious mind.

Let me restate that your subconscious mind is 90% of your mind, and your conscious mind is only 10% or less. You have been using only 10% of your mind's power to achieve your goal. Through hypnosis, self-hypnosis, meditation and/or mindfulness, you can harness the power of your subconscious mind, and approach weight loss with 100% of your mind.

Understanding how you get fat is helpful in fighting the

'dis-ease' of being overweight. This book will educate you in easy-to-understand terms: the interaction of hypnosis, your mind, homeostasis, nutrition, toxins, inflammation, neurochemicals, emotions, habits, neuroplasticity, stress, anxiety, sense of purpose, obesogens, body syndromes, subconscious desires, vibrational levels and the importance of sleep.

In most cases, this information is included because of its direct impact on weight loss or weight gain. In some cases, however, there is an indirect impact. Indirect impacts can include the need to feel happy and fulfilled, and to have the confidence and self-esteem that will motivate you to maintain this new lifestyle.

Of course, you want to be healthy, live a long and productive life. That is a given. But how you feel in your own skin is often just as important to your well-being (and affects your overall health) as well. We will cover all of this, and you will walk away with knowledge and tools that can be applied to many other aspects of your life.

The mechanics of weight gain and weight loss are primarily discussed in the first part of the book, and the focus is on changing your mindset and subconscious programming. Chapters 1 to 7 focus on the power of the mind, why you gain weight, how you can perform self-hypnosis to implement all of this new information and reprogram your mind for success.

Chapters 8 to 11 explain metabolism, the gut-biome, nutrition, exercise and sleep. The book explains why these are critical for successful weight maintenance, and what you need to do to achieve this.

THIS IS THE LAST DIET BOOK YOU WILL EVER HAVE TO READ. ONCE YOU HAVE 'UPGRADED YOUR SOFTWARE' MEANING CHANGED YOUR PAST PROGRAMMING WITH THE KNOWLEDGE CONTAINED IN THIS BOOK, YOU WILL BE EMPOWERED TO MAKE LASTING AND IMPACTFUL CHANGES IN YOUR LIFE. THIS WILL LEAD TO AUTOMATIC AND SUSTAINED WEIGHT LOSS, AND STABLE WEIGHT MANAGEMENT THEREAFTER.

Chapter 2: Your Incredible Mind

Let's begin by gaining a basic understanding of how our minds work. As mentioned previously, losing weight is all about harnessing the power of your subconscious mind. The following diagram is known as 'Theory of Mind'. It looks complicated, but once you come to understand how the mind works, it will make much more sense to you.

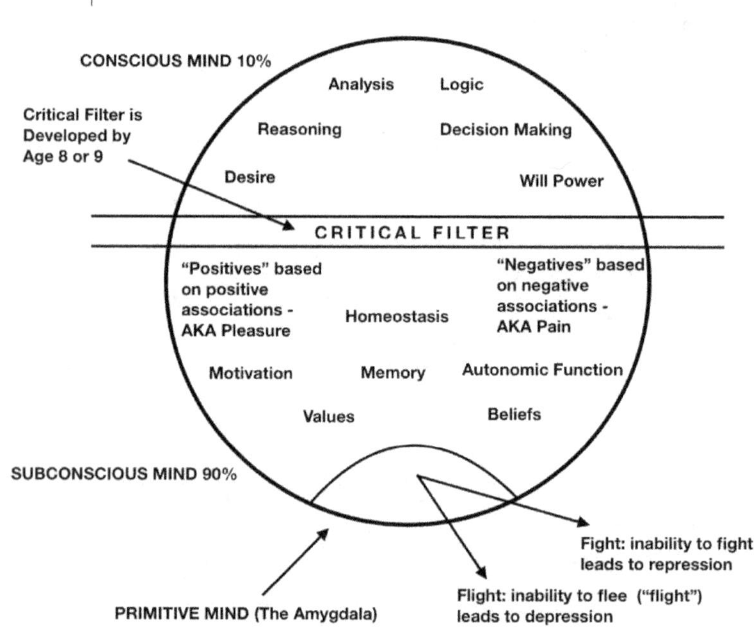

Follow the diagram as I explain it:

1. Your mind consists of two main parts: the conscious and subconscious.
2. The conscious mind makes up about 10% of your mind. It is responsible for elements such as logic, analysis, reasoning, willpower and decision making.
3. Your subconscious mind makes up about 90% of your mind. It is responsible for all of your body's functions that you are unaware of consciously, such as your blood pumping and digestion.
4. The subconscious also handles elements such as emotions, motivation, values, and beliefs.
5. Your subconscious mind is fully programmed by age eight. Your programming comes from your life experiences, associations, events, physiology, behavior and the role models in your life (especially your parents).
6. When you are born, you have a wide-eyed innocence. Then you start to realize that things are not always as they seem. You start to develop a critical filter (also called the analytical filter) as you age, and by the age of eight or nine this filter has fully developed. Before this, children take in information literally and have no filter with which to judge what they are told, what they see, or what they experience.
7. Before eight and after, we form associations with things, both positive and negative. Perhaps a dog bit you at age 6 and you are still terrified of dogs at age 20. Or you had a wonderful dog in childhood, and you've always loved dogs. We associate things as

being good, bad, known or unknown. And we keep those associations intact unless something changes them (such as hypnosis). Left unchanged, when we experience a similar circumstance later in life, that old association comes up again, and we react in the way we reacted the first time, generally as a child. As opposed to responding with the adult lens of reasoning; analysis; logic; decision-making; and will power. When a fact or suggestion is presented to you, the critical filter acts as a gateway to your subconscious mind. If the fact **does not** fit with your version of the world, then this fact or suggestion is rejected; if it **does** fit with you know to be true, then this fact or suggestion is accepted by your conscious and subconscious minds.

8. Within your subconscious mind is a part known as the primitive mind. Physically, this sits in a part of the brain called the amygdala. The primitive mind is responsible for protecting the animal entity (You) through a threat response mechanism. When confronted with a threat, the primitive mind automatically generates a sympathetic nervous system response of fight-or-flight. Your mind instantly assesses the risk and decides whether to fight or run away. Physiologically the response is the same: neuro-hormones such as cortisol and adrenaline are pumped into your body to enable a rapid response, and blood is pumped away from the organs and into the limbs, to enable fight or flight.

9. Your experiences and associations starting at birth are the conditioning which formed your fears, values, beliefs, morals, and capabilities. These created the

script in your subconscious mind. Your success in life is dependent on the constraints contained in that script.

10. The subconscious mind's primary function is survival. Any unknowns are seen as a potential threat. To the subconscious mind, staying the same (the 'known') equates to safety. No matter how desirable the 'unknown' may be (such as a newly trim body), it is unfamiliar and is thus perceived as a threat.

11. As mentioned, homeostasis (staying the same; the norm, or set-point) is your current state (your known). If your current situation is an overweight state, we need to change your programming, so that what you envision to be a perfect weight becomes your new level of homeostasis (your known). If your homeostasis is programmed to be that you are currently lean, your subconscious mind will make sure that the body is congruent (or in agreement) with that. And that is what you will become...and how you will stay.

12. We as humans are biologically programmed to seek pleasure and to avoid pain. The avoidance of pain is stronger than the seeking of pleasure because pain could mean a threat to survival. If a caveman ate a poisonous berry and became very ill, he needed to remember to avoid those berries in the future. This is more important than remembering the pleasurable tasting peach he found the day before. Thus, we as humans 1) like things to stay the same (homeostasis); 2) avoid things for which we have developed negative associations with (avoiding pain), and 3) seek things for which we have positive associations with (seeking

pleasure).

13. The goal of this book is first, to help you reprogram your subconscious mind in order to change unwanted behavior. The most powerful route to do this is to understand how your mind works and its biological motivations. Reprogramming your subconscious script so that the image of you at your perfect weight is implanted into your subconscious mind. Second, we need to change 'dislikes' to 'likes.' You can start liking foods that you did not, as well as liking (and looking forward to) exercise and other healthy activities.

14. Your subconscious mind is a goal-seeking machine. When it has a mission, it will manifest things in your life that will move you to this goal. Some of these things will be physical (food, exercise, sleep). Others will be metaphysical (for instance, through some sort of 'divine intervention' you might end up at yoga, which you never thought possible). It does not matter because the end (results) justify the means.

15. Quantum physics has proven that YOU create YOUR world. But your world is only what is programmed into your subconscious. Allow yourself to reprogram your subconscious mind with everything you desire in 'your version' of a perfect world.

After reprogramming yourself (through self-hypnosis, mindfulness, meditation, and other methods described later in this book), this process will become automatic and unstoppable. You will achieve your desired outcome. Many people, after hypnosis, meet their intended goals and then decide that hypnosis is not necessary and did not facilitate the change. That is because the new goal is now programmed into their subconscious mind and they 'own' it.   It comes from within them. It is their new 'known'. This change becomes a new lifestyle, which creates a slimmer, happier version of you.

You do not have to use hypnosis to reprogram your mind. There are other ways to do it. Mindfulness and meditation are very useful tools for changing values inside your mind as well. But hypnosis and self-hypnosis can accelerate the process.

Later in the book, I will teach you how to do self-hypnosis, which is a powerful tool to bring positive changes into your life. Right now, you may wish to focus on weight loss, and when you see how effective it is, you may decide to use it for other things such as happiness, wealth, relationships, and career. Once your self-confidence and well-being are transformed, you may want to change anything else standing in your way to true joy and fulfillment.

Chapter 3: Your Incredible Body

Let's learn a little about what makes us tick.

Chemicals

Did you realize you were a chemical addict? As human beings, we are simple creatures. We are driven by chemicals, hormones, and neurotransmitters, which are continually being released into the body. The acronym D.O.S.E. describes the 4 chemicals our body craves. They are Dopamine, Oxytocin, Serotonin, and Endorphins.

'Positive' Chemicals	Mind Link
Dopamine	A Feeling of Success
Oxytocin	A Feeling of Trust
Serotonin	A Feeling of Importance
Endorphins	A Feeling of Euphoria

At our lowest level, our body is made up of chemical elements with some electricity. At a level slightly further up, we are simply reptilian animals, whose behavior is driven by the addiction to those four chemicals—and others such as acetylcholine and GABA. We are programmed to continually seek out and fulfill a chemical 'fix.'

Through a feel-good chemical release, the brain's pleasure center knows when something is enjoyable, which reinforces the desire for us to repeat that pleasurable action. This is called the 'reward circuit' and includes all pleasure, from sex to laughter, to certain types of drug use. As the brain perceives pleasure, it impacts the body in various ways:

- **Amygdala** - Regulates Emotions.
- **Nucleus Accumbens** - Controls the Release of Dopamine.
- **Ventral Tegmental Area (VTA)** – Releases the Dopamine.
- **Cerebellum** – Controls Muscle Function.
- **Pituitary Gland** – Releases:
    - Beta-Endorphins (which decrease pain)
    - Oxytocin (which increases feelings of trust)
    - Vasopressin (which increases bonding)

These chemicals have evolutionary functions—for instance, sex ensures the procreation of all species, bonding ensures our young are cared for, etc. Because we crave the stimulus of these chemicals, our value system is affected. We evaluate the actions we take in relation to the type and amount of chemical released by that particular action. Often the chemical release determines whether we like something or we don't. In effect, we are rewarding ourselves with chemicals for activities/actions that we then determine the value/priority of. This is all about you—nothing external has interfered with this process. It is all taking place within what I call our 'mindbody' (because they are truly one system).

This is why hypnotherapy is so successful. With hypnosis,

you are able to reprioritize and to reassign values to activities/actions. In short, you can learn new behaviors and assign an appropriate chemical release to reinforce the perceived value of this new behavior.

The feel-good chemicals are perceived as pleasure, and the feel-bad chemicals (like cortisol) are perceived as pain. Chemicals like acetylcholine lead to relaxation, which stimulates our reward center, and is thus perceived by our mindbody as good. Chemicals like epinephrine and norepinephrine stimulate the sympathetic nervous system, lead to a heightened state—such as fight-or-flight, fear and anxiety—and are perceived by the reward center as 'bad.'

An absence of feel-good chemicals leaves us uneasy, and we are programmed to achieve the release of them. At a base level, this is nothing more than a teaching process, where our behavior becomes Pavlovian (or stemming from basic classical conditioning). Our 'path,' is driven by the subconscious according to a predetermined set of rules: of seeking out the 'good' and avoiding the 'bad.'

If we have established values for certain things, and our mind releases 'feel-good' chemicals as a reward for fulfilling these values, then it stands to reason that we can reprogram our mind, to install different motivational programs. The reprogramming part takes a bit of practice, but mostly what you need is a desire and willingness to change. The rest becomes automatic.

Brainwave States

Every second of the day, each neuron and synapse in our brain is firing with electrical energy. We measure this cyclical energy in Hertz (cycles per second) which depict the varying frequencies of electrical energy within our brains. We call these 'brainwave states.'

Some Examples of Brainwave States:

- **Delta (0.5 Hz to 4 Hz):** When the body is in its deepest sleep, healing, and rejuvenating itself. Generally, a person is unconscious in this state. A person in a coma would be in a delta state. Drugs or other substances can also induce it.
- **Theta (4 Hz to 7.5 Hz):** Light (REM) sleep, dreaming and deep meditation. A person in theta can also experience a deep connection to source, profound insights, and visualizations. Light sleep, deep hypnosis, emotions such as gratitude.
- **Alpha (7.5 Hz to 12.5 Hz):** When we are very relaxed, about to drift off to sleep, daydreaming, traveling without consciously remembering the route. It is also associated with intuitive thinking, insight, creativity, and deep relaxation.
- **Beta (12.5 Hz to 30 Hz):** Typical state when we are awake, and our general mental awareness when actively engaged in the world. In this state, the physical senses are alert and actively taking in information.
- **Gamma (30 Hz to 60 Hz):** Associated with higher mental functioning, anxiety, extreme excitement,

euphoria, being 'in the zone' and peak concentration. Also fight-or-flight, terror, and shock.

As we go through life, we are constantly bombarded with stimuli and millions of bits of information (we will refer to as 'message units') from our external and internal world. We need to process these message units, store what we need, discard what we don't and start over again. We do this sort of 'clean-up process' during REM sleep.

Our brains operate at different wavelengths depending on our state, emotions, nutrition, and external factors. The higher the brainwave state, the more message units we take in. This constant influx of information must be processed to make room for more, or we become overloaded and overwhelmed.

For instance, we can only be in a gamma range for a short time before we are overloaded (such as an athlete's ability to run a long distance slowly, but short distances at high speed). Gamma is high speed, so it generates a significant number of message units. Anxiety is a gamma state, so people in anxiety are giving themselves a more massive dose of message units every day. This is the reason some people have nervous breakdowns, or have psychotic attacks—the mind simply cannot cope with the continuous high volume of message units.

Conversely, because of the relaxed state of our bodies at lower Hertz levels, fewer message units are created and received, and we are also better able to cope with stored message units. This is perceived by the mind as relaxation.

In REM sleep and deep sleep, the mind begins to purge itself of message units. It also achieves this through the neuro-linguistic programming (NLP) processes of delete, distort and generalizing data, but unwanted thoughts and message units are mostly vented out through dreams. Think of the analogy of the brain as a computer hard disk—during the day it gets full, and at night it is emptied to create storage space. So an anxious person will find it difficult to achieve relaxation, and even more difficult to achieve sleep. The net effect is that the message units are not removed, more are taken in, and the anxiety increases. This becomes a vicious spiral.

Hypnosis is a state of mind that allows us to temporarily bypass our critical filter (analytical mind) and allow reprogramming of our beliefs, motivations, and values. In this altered state, we open up a gateway to the subconscious where these programs reside. Ordinarily, the critical mind is the gatekeeper of the subconscious mind and has a strict set of rules. Hypnosis bypasses these rules and allows manipulation of the subconscious mind. Through hypnosis or self-hypnosis, we can access our subconscious mind and reprogram it so that it contains the elements of our life that we desire – such as a lean, slim, muscular body.

Chapter 4: Weight Loss and the Mind

Obesity is a disease with deadly consequences. In 1975 the average American's daily calorie intake was 3,100 calories. In 2000, it was over 4,000 calories. Our annual sugar intake has also increased exponentially every year.

Hypnosis/mindfulness/meditation are all very effective in assisting weight loss. When you decide to diet, you approach it with your conscious mind and not your subconscious mind. So, if the conscious mind is 10% of your mind, and the subconscious makes up 90%, you have an uphill battle.

You may set out with good intentions to exercise more and make better food choices. But your subconscious mind is not on board and sees any change as a potential threat. Thus, it will continually sabotage your mission. If only 10% of your mind is committed to your diet goals: then the other 90% will be committed to subverting them.

Let me give you a simplistic example: as a kid, when you were good, Mom gave you candy. When things were rough (for instance a pet died), then Mom gave you candy. When you fell off your bike, Mom patched you up and gave you candy. So the subconscious mind has a positive association with candy—and here you are trying to give it up. To get the subconscious mind on board with your diet, we need to reprogram the subconscious mind's associations. For instance, the association of linking candy to feeling good can be 'dis-associated.' Once this reprogramming has taken root, giving up candy (or its equivalent) will be a whole lot easier.

For as long as you try to give up candy while the subconscious sees it as a positive, you are depriving yourself. And the subconscious mind does not do deprivation. Its primary role is to protect you, and deprivation of any kind is not seen as protecting you. The subconscious has formed associations with food, and some of these are sustenance, nutrition, satiety, and happiness. Your subconscious will not easily allow you to deprive yourself of these. And as your subconscious is the most powerful part of your mind, you will ultimately not win this battle. That is unless you can convince your subconscious of two things: first to let go of the 'survival' associations with food (nutrition, satiety, etc.), and second to convince the subconscious of the benefits of weight loss (health, esthetics, etc.). With the latter aspect, a healthy person has a better chance of survival—and when this fact registers to the subconscious, it becomes the subconscious' primary task.

The primary reason hypnotherapy is so successful in weight loss is that we enable the subconscious mind to accept our new image of ourselves. The second reason is this: in most cases a person who is overweight got there because of an emotional cause. When they diet, they are only treating the symptom and not the cause.

Hypnotherapy can treat the cause, and neutralize it, thus enabling a successful weight loss program and ensuring that any weight lost, does not return at a later date.

The 6 Pillars of Weight Loss™

I founded a company called Thinessence™, because I believe that weight loss is a holistic process that involves both mind and body. It is the first hypnosis weight loss and wellness clinic of its kind. We use several modalities in addition to hypnotherapy, all centered around what we call the 6 Pillars of Weight Loss™. Those are:

- Hypnosis
- Entrainment (brain entrainment)
- Nutrition
- Emotional Aspects
- Lifestyle Changes
- Homeostasis

The point is this: hypnotherapy on its own can be very effective. But when combined with other facets such as exercise, nutrition, stress reduction, and tools such as The Emotional Freedom Technique (or 'EFT'), and other therapeutic modalities, it becomes increasingly powerful. See **www.thinessence.com** for details about other modalities that can be applied to weight loss success. Here is a brief description of these elements, some of which are discussed in detail further in the book.

Homeostasis

We stay within the parameters of our subconscious script, which is our 'known'. So, if our script is programmed that we are overweight, we will remain overweight no matter what we do. Change is perceived as a potential threat and is avoided by the subconscious mind.

Body Syndromes

Where on the body is the weight carried? Using a theory called 'Body Syndromes,' can help us pinpoint the reason for my unwanted weight. And how easily it can be let go. For instance, pain in certain areas can depict certain emotional traumas, such as pain in shoulders can relate to the stress of responsibilities weighing heavily on one's shoulders, or a sore throat can mean holding back speaking your mind. The accumulation of body fat is often linked to being oversensitive (either in general or to a particular issue, e.g. sexual image). Typically, a person is overweight for one of two reasons: an emotional cause, or an addiction to neurochemicals—like eating bread or sugar to get a serotonin and dopamine release. Body Syndromes are discussed in detail in the next Chapter.

Expectations

A person might expect drastic weight loss, and then lose motivation when it does not happen. With hypnotherapy, weight loss is an automatic function of reprogramming; but the most important aspect is inducing a lifestyle change. A weight loss of 1lb per week is healthy and sustainable. Should you exceed this loss, you are welcome to get excited, but keep in mind that the slower the loss, the more permanent the results. With a fad diet, weight loss can be extreme, but it is like a pendulum—the quicker you lose it, the quicker you gain it back (and sometimes even more).

The lifestyle changes brought about through hypnotherapy are exactly that—lifestyle changes. Excess weight will gradually be shed until a stable or goal weight is reached, and then it will plateau at that level. Remember, of course, that your homeostasis has to be adjusted so that your subconscious accepts this new weight level as your norm.

What You Think is What You Become/Affirmations

Our thoughts are very powerful: as you think, so shall you become. Be aware of the quality of your thoughts; if those thoughts are focused on the excessive weight, unhappiness, need for overeating, then your thoughts are working against you. Visualize yourself at your goal weight as if this is the case today, and have all of your thoughts support this. Customize daily affirmations to suit your situation and say the affirmations several times a day. Make them positive and in the present tense. Such as 'I am thin and toned'; 'I only desire foods that nourish my body'; I love what I look like in clothes'; I feel confident in my own skin,' etc.

Never think about the act of losing the weight and what needs to be changed. Think of who you will be at the end of it and how you will feel. Use your senses to intensify this, by imagining your perfect body image in a scene, maybe sitting at a sidewalk café in Paris, or walking through Central Park in New York. Or maybe at a party with admiring friends. Use your imagination. Once you lock in the location, add in what you are wearing, how your hair looks, possibly the fragrance you have on, the time of day or night, who is there, what they are doing, and every possible detail. Hear the sounds you would hear, smell the smells you would smell, taste the flavors you would taste, feel the feelings you would *feel*. Really experience these visualizations with as many of your senses as possible to lock them into your subconscious programming. Your subconscious mind cannot discern the difference between reality and imagination, and with repetition, this can be a powerful tool in your arsenal.

Hollywood actress Alexis Smith once quoted, 'Positive thinking works beautifully on a reducing diet. Never think once about what you are giving up, but concentrate on what you are getting.'

Emotional Intelligence

You are overweight for a reason. Chances are you do not recognize what that reason is. Consciously you desire to be thin. Subconsciously your mind sees you as overweight and is not interested in making any changes. Therefore, it sends signals for you to do things that do not support the conscious choice you've made to lose weight. Until you have rectified this anomaly, you will remain overweight. Your 'Emotional Intelligence' is a scale of the connection you have to your mindbody, it is a measure of how much you listen to your mindbody and take action when the mindbody sends you a signal. Some of us are not connected to our mindbody; thus, we have low Emotional

Intelligence.

Hypnosis helps reduce the conscious 'noise' so that we can begin a dialogue with our subconscious mind (SCM); over time, continued dialogue helps to improve our connection to the SCM, and thereby increases our Emotional Intelligence. You can diet as much as you like but you are only addressing the symptom. A diet will not be a permanent 'fix' until you have rectified **the cause** of you being overweight. Ask your subconscious why it thinks you should be overweight. Agree to let it go and accept the new image of you.

**Law of Concentrated Attention
(Law of Belief/Probability/Repetition)**

As previously mentioned, the subconscious is a goal-seeking machine. A particular function or event (for instance a wedding, high school reunion, graduation, or Uncle Pete's 50th birthday party) for which you desire to slim down for, acts as a very useful target and tool. For instance, select a picture of a slim person wearing a sexy outfit and this now becomes your new image. Save it as your screensaver on your computer, your mobile phone, and even print out copies and put them on your bathroom mirror, desk at work, etc. Start to believe that this is the new you – one way to reprogram your subconscious is repetition.

Keep sending this image to your subconscious, and soon enough your subconscious will adopt this image as being the real you. It will then move heaven and earth to ensure this transpires.

Mindfulness and Gratitude

These are powerful tools in weight loss and are discussed later.

Stress Reduction

When we are under stress, our bodies create a set of 'negative' neurohormones which include cortisol, epinephrine, and norepinephrine.

> **Norepinephrine**: tells our body to stop producing insulin so that plenty of fast-acting blood glucose is ready when we need it.

> **Epinephrine:** relaxes the muscles in our stomach and intestines and decreases blood flow to these organs.

> **Cortisol:** takes fat from healthier areas, like the buttocks and hips, and moves it to the abdomen which has more cortisol receptors, increasing inflammation and insulin resistance in the body. This creates a vicious circle—belly fat then leads to more cortisol because it has higher concentrations of an enzyme that converts inactive cortisone to active cortisol. The more belly fat we have, the more active cortisol will be converted by these enzymes. When our stress and cortisol levels are high, the body resists

weight loss.

Subconscious Blocks

Right this moment, in your mind, define your ideal weight and picture yourself at that weight. Now pause, focus on your body and mind, and acknowledge the negative signals now presenting themselves. For instance, perhaps the feedback you are getting is 'there is no way I can look like that,' or 'that seems like depriving myself for a long time.' Consider these 'negative' statements.

If possible, rationalize what the negative statements are, where they came from, and whether you can start releasing them. Replace these negative thoughts with positive thoughts. These are your subconscious blocks to losing weight.

Chapter 5: Body Syndromes

The location of where the adipose tissue (what you may call 'fat') has accumulated on your body is an indication of how it got there. Men and women typically have different 'fat patterns'. - Men typically display 'android' fat distribution patterns, and women 'gynoid'. Usually, a person is obese for one of two reasons: an emotional cause, or an addiction to neurochemicals—like eating bread or sugar to get a serotonin and dopamine release.

Another aspect of body syndromes is hormones; where possible, hormones should be in balance. When the hormones are not in balance, this will cause certain organs (e.g. the thyroid) to malfunction, leading to an over-production or under-production of hormones or enzymes. This, in turn, leads to excess weight being deposited in a specific area of the body. For instance, excess estrogen in men often leads to the formation of male breasts ('man boobs'). Knowing what body type you are is an indication of what possible hormone imbalance you have, and therefore how it might be rectified.

Consider the following weight-related body shapes and origins of adipose tissue:

Body Shape	Cause
1 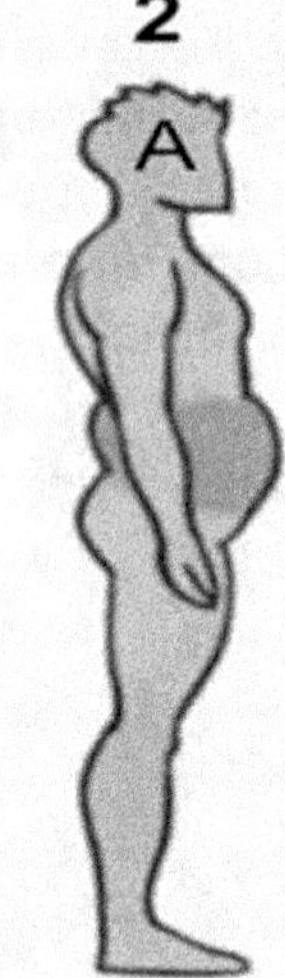	**Upper Body Syndrome (Android)** This body type is typical of a person who overeats and exercises too little. It is also typical of a person with a poor gut biome, heavily dependent on sugar, alcohol and fast food. Also displayed by diabetics, and people who used to exercise a lot, and those who have poor metabolism. This body type usually has high estrogen, low testosterone, high cortisol and high insulin levels Solution: less sugar, more probiotics, healthy food, more fiber, more exercise. Less stress.
2	**Waistline Syndrome (Android)** This body type is typical of a person who has hormonal issues and too much cortisol release. The cortisol is probably stress-related. This is also indicative of a person with a sedentary lifestyle, and who sits too much – perhaps a deskbound person or truck driver. Excess sugar or alcohol is also a culprit. This body type usually has high estrogen and testosterone levels, and high cortisol levels. Solution: healthy food, more fiber, more exercise. Less sitting.

3  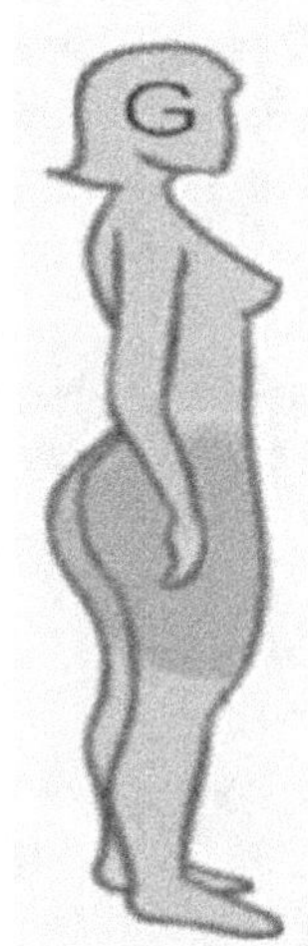	**Lower Body Syndrome (Gynoid)** Hormonal issues, menopause, and genetics are typically responsible for this body type. Also, women sensitive to gluten display this body shape. This body type usually has high estrogen, low progesterone, and low growth hormone levels. Solution: healthy food, more fiber, more aerobic exercise like walking. Reduce all foods containing gluten.
4  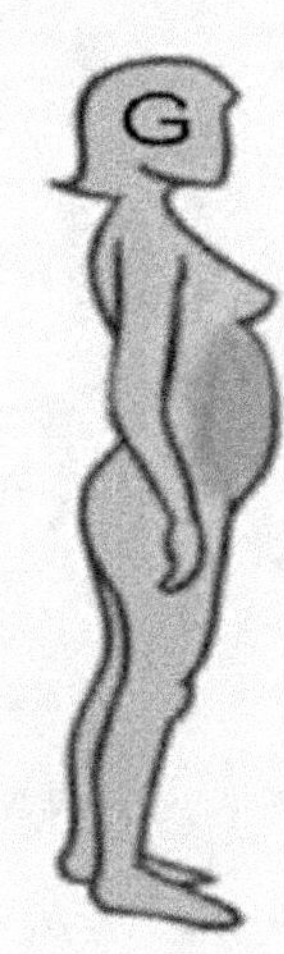	**Protruding Stomach (Gynoid)** A protruding stomach is typical of food allergies, over-consumption of the same food types, fast-food, sugar, alcohol, wheat and inflammation caused by the wrong foods. People who do not breathe deeply also display this body shape. It is also indicative of stress and suppressed emotional issues. This body type usually has high testosterone and cortisol levels. Solution: healthy food, more fiber, zero gluten, more aerobic exercise. Breathing exercises, yoga, hypnosis.

5	Leg Syndrome (Gynoid)
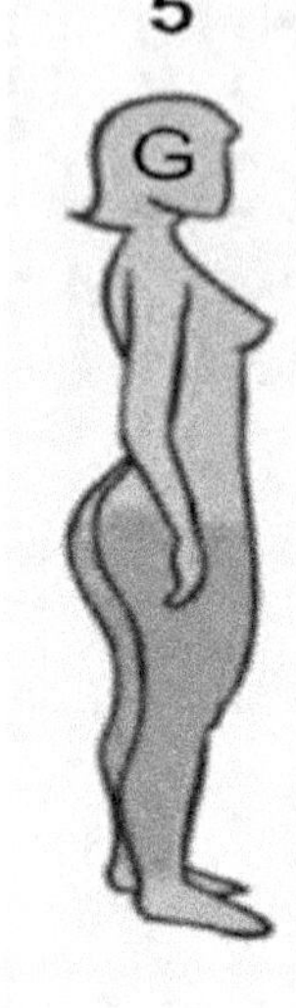	Genetics, hormonal issues or pregnancy are a typical cause of this body type. Water retention and poor circulation can also be responsible. This body type usually has high estrogen, low progesterone and low growth hormone levels. Solution: healthy food, zero gluten, more aerobic exercise. More water and less salt. Breathing exercises. Yoga.

Chapter 6: Re-Program Your Mind

We are all born with a script. This is a summation of our experiences, values, and beliefs. Typically, we will stay within the parameters of the script we have been programmed with. Yet we have an amazing ability to rewrite that script, to increase our worthiness, our expectations and achieve what we desire. There are proven ways to increase our success, prosperity and happiness. This is such an important concept that I have restated it throughout the book.

Henry Ford said, 'Whether you think you can, or think you can't, you are right.' This statement is brilliant in its simplicity and underlines the creative power we all have. The quote is wrong in one area. 'Think you can' implies it is a conjecture of the conscious mind. Change this to 'know you can.' When the subconscious mind accepts something as real, it will manifest that reality.

The Power of Thought

Everything about you is electromagnetic. Each cell in your body, each organ, fiber, vessel, muscle and bone has an electromagnetic vibration. Your brain has a high electromagnetic vibration, only surpassed by your heart. Each thought you think has an electromagnetic vibration, as does every word you say.

Anything with electromagnetic qualities has an 'attracting' force. Each of your thoughts attracts or repels events and experiences in line with your vibration level.

Who you are, how you think, and how you act all create the manifestation that you attract.

Only twenty years ago researchers learned that the hypothalamus transforms a thought or mental image into millions of neuropeptides that represent the emotion of that thought. For every experience of thought, the brain's 'control center' releases a storm of amino acids into the bloodstream, which then insert themselves into cells within the brain-body system. And, over time, these cells begin to crave these particular neuropeptides, creating a self-fulfilling prophecy of emotion. Now, scientists find that negative thoughts not only affect mood but also other aspects of physical health. Increasing levels of inflammation in the body are associated with a number of disorders and conditions.

Energy carries information. Recent studies prove that water flowing in a river had more information at the river mouth than at its source. Somehow it had ''acquired' information along the way. So, your thoughts have powerful information which you transfer to your body (and the Universe). It is a two-way street—everything you come into contact with transfers information to you, and you to it.

Think of your subconscious mind as a bank – whatever you deposit will grow, and will earn compound interest. Deposit thoughts of prosperity, wealth, success, love, joy, and gratitude. And know that when you have thoughts of fear, anger, doubt, anxiety – then you are making a withdrawal from your account.

It may take some time to realize the impact of your thinking. But once you grasp it, and start to implement more positive thinking, you will find that your world becomes rapidly and positively transformed. What you think, you become.

Quantum physics says that you, the Observer, create reality from chaos. You, the Observer, are the Creator of your world, your universe. You probably try your best with everything you do in life. Knowing the power you possess, why not choose to create a perfect existence?

Self-Hypnosis

Self-hypnosis is an easy, effective, and often transformational tool. You are where you are today because of the series of decisions you have made. Self-hypnosis allows you to take charge of things you want to change and re-create your life. Customizing your life to match your desires and intentions. Once you've made those decisions to change, self-hypnosis allows you to make better choices and behave in ways, that facilitate your new reality.

I will take you step by step, through learning to use self-hypnosis to program the 'new you' for weight loss and once you have mastered it, you can begin to use it in other areas of your life that you may want to improve upon. What you will be doing is reprogramming your mind to associate certain forms of stimuli to positive, calm feelings rather than negative, anxious ones and vice versa.

Contract with Self

You only have your motivation to lose weight. For some people, this is not enough. See the Appendix for a Weight Loss Contract. Fill in the contract, sign it – it is now a binding contract with your subconscious mind.

Homeostasis

Your subconscious mindset of who you are will dictate whether or not you remain lean or return to your former state. According to the concept of homeostasis, if you believe you are poor, you will remain poor. Similarly, if you believe you are fat, you will remain fat.

Program your mind to:

- Start to see your body as an expensive sports car, with a powerful engine. Every day you need a large amount of quality food for your quality engine.
- Visualize your cells at a higher metabolic rate. Picture yourself having a 'fat thermostat' – and turn it down to its lowest possible level.
- Picture the best version of you. I call this '[insert your name here] Version 2.0' – imagine your body, but as version 2.0, make the image larger, more detailed, more definition, more color. Now give the image a burst of feel-good energy.
- Imagine how you feel when you become this new you. Use the intensity of that feeling to power the

image and burn it into your subconscious, many times a day.

- Homeostasis is the desire to stay the same. The subconscious mind hates unknowns, and our inherent efficiency keeps us using the same neural pathways. Much of what we do every day is in a form of autopilot. We are thinking and doing the same thing we did yesterday...and the day before that...and the year before that. We stick to the same habits, routines, and patterns and avoid change. This keeps us 'stuck' at the level of our script.

A person who is programmed to believe they receive love/attention/sympathy only when they are a victim (or poor, or depressed, or ill...) will have a hard time changing to a successful person (or wealthy, or happy, or healthy...). In order to change your level of homeostasis in any particular category, you can harness five tools:

1. Be open to all possibilities, and allow yourself to set the bar higher, dream of bigger things, have a sense of self-worth, and come to 'believe' in the new script.
2. Use daily reinforcement of all the tools and tips described here. The primary law of 'suggestibility' (which is to accept information into your subconscious mind as truth) is repetition.
3. Your brain works with symbolic language. For instance, you can use the $ (dollar) symbol not only to indicate wealth and abundance, but also as a symbol to signify your increased joy, love, peace, etc.
4. Handwriting (which is discussed further on)

5. Pick a specific time of day to manifest your new reality, to do your affirmations, do the Mental Bank (which we will detail later in the book), and/or to practice gratitude. A good time to do this is just before sleep—because of the alpha brainwave state (the frequency of brain waves which we will discuss in a later chapter) you drift into, the gate to your subconscious is already open.

Affirmations

...I love myself. I love my life...

...My body knows what is good for it
and seeks those foods...

...Every day in every way I am lighter and lighter, thinner and thinner, happier and happier...

These are examples of affirmations, but they can come in hundreds of thousands of different varieties that you create with words that have specific meaning to you.

Using positive affirmations daily help you to:

- vibrate at a higher level (we are made of energy)
- attract the outcome you are describing
- start to move you up the emotional spiral
- focus on what you desire in life
- get into a state of gratitude

An affirmation is a carefully formatted statement that should be written down and repeated to oneself

---

frequently. For an affirmation to be effective, it needs to be:

- Present Tense
- Positive
- Personal
- Specific

The subconscious mind does not know the difference between real or imagined, positive or negative. So do not say for instance: 'I **don't** want to eat cake' because your mind will only hear 'I want to eat cake'. Also, say things in the present tense. Instead of saying 'I will be thin' which is in the future-tense, say 'I am thin'. Most importantly it should include an inclusion of **gratitude**. Gratitude is the highest form of the present tense, as it is saying that you are grateful for something that you already have now.

The word affirmation comes from the Latin *affirmare*, originally meaning 'to make steady, to strengthen.' And that is what it does to our lives—it steadies and strengthens us, our mind, our body, and our beliefs.

Affirmations are proven methods of self-improvement because of their ability to rewire our brains. Much like exercise, they raise the level of feel-good hormones and push our brains to form new clusters of 'positive thought' neurons (see: **http://arlenetaylor.org/brain-care/953-affirmation** for more detail). In the sequence of thought-speech-action, affirmations play an integral role by breaking patterns of negative thoughts, negative speech, and, in turn, negative actions.

The most powerful affirmations are those that create images in the subconscious. As you state your affirmation VISUALIZE the end result in your mind.

See yourself as **being** 25lbs lighter, see you **driving** your new car, **picture** the check for a million dollars written to you (in detail – who is the check from? Date? Signed by?). The subconscious mind works in symbols and images, not language. You need to affirm in symbols and images.

Repeat your affirmation often enough that it becomes a mantra of your life. Be as specific as you can, and truly **believe** in the affirmation. It is your unwavering belief in the words that bring about the manifestation. Without belief, affirmations are just empty words. And the law of repetition says that continual exposure to something makes it a 'truth' over time.

Dr. Bruce Lipton (see, '7 Ways to Reprogram Your Mind') states, 'Your subconscious beliefs are working either for you or against you, but the truth is that you are not controlling your life, because your subconscious mind supersedes all conscious control. So when you are trying to heal from a conscious level—citing affirmations and telling yourself you're healthy—there may be an invisible subconscious program that's sabotaging you.'

A list of resources to find affirmations along with instructions on how best to use them can be found in the appendix.

Chapter 7: The Self-Hypnosis Process

Understanding Why You are Overweight

Before you start the self-hypnosis process, it helps to understand why you might be overweight. Being as honest as possible, consider the following questions and attempt a deep understanding of the answer that presents itself. At first, an answer might seem strange, even unacceptable. Allow the answer, and then ponder possible ramifications of the answer. Feel the answers within your body and see what comes up. You will use these truths for the following hypnotic process.

Twelve questions for change:

1. Why do you want to lose weight?
2. Why have you been unable to lose weight, or maintain weight, in the past?
3. What are the things causing stress in your life right now?
4. What are the emotional reasons you are overeating?
5. Food is a substitute. What are you really actually hungry for?
6. What are your negative beliefs about losing weight?
7. Do you have any fears about losing weight?
8. What issues from the past still affect you?
9. If you were bored, feeling down or stressed, instead of eating, what enjoyable thing can you do?
10. What are all the benefits of, and reasons for, losing weight?

11. What are the positive feelings and emotions you would have if you were your ideal weight?
12. What are the emotional reasons you want to lose weight?

Consider your conscious AND subconscious responses to these questions. A good reason might present itself as to why you have not been able to lose weight permanently. Alternatively, a subconscious reason might present itself. Analyze this to see the best way you can change any negative to a positive. Finally, using self-hypnosis, reprogram your subconscious mind so that all the new positives are coded into the core of who you are.

The Self-Hypnosis Process

When you first start doing self-hypnosis, you may feel a little self-conscious. All it takes is a bit of perseverance and practice. If you get stuck on any step, skip that step, and go to the next one. Next time around, try and include the skipped step. In a short period of time, you will have mastered self-hypnosis.

There are many methods to induce self-hypnosis. We are all different, and over time each of us will adopt a method that suits us best. This section details a self-hypnosis 'induction' (which means the process of getting you into a hypnotic state) that works well for me and my clients. In the next section, I include several other methods, which you might prefer. Try them all and see what works for you.

Preferably find a time and place where you will not be disturbed. You can be sitting in a comfortable chair, or lying in bed at night, or even when you wake up. Make sure you are comfortable, with minimal distractions. Any breathing exercises you may already know how to use, can help relax you, and bring you to an alpha state, meaning slow down your brainwaves to more easily enter a hypnotic state.

With self-hypnosis, your mind will have a tendency to drift—do not try to control this, but rather allow this expansion of the mind. After you have 'wandered' a little, gently bring your attention back to the process. Self-hypnosis is an amazing tool for self-discovery, and sometimes people may experience revelations.

Preparation

Bedtime is always a good time for self-hypnosis, because the body is producing melatonin and preparing to shut down, in readiness for the sleep process. Avoid stimulants from the afternoon onwards, and try to avoid too much screen time with electronic devices. Develop a nighttime ritual such as having a bath with essential oils. Or maybe a cup of chamomile tea to help you relax.

Once in bed, perhaps you might read a book or write in a journal to wind down further. The point in which you are ready to switch out the light and go to sleep, is the optimum time for self-hypnosis (because of the naturally-occurring slower alpha brainwave state).

Many people think that going into hypnosis 'gives up' their power of self-control for a period of time. This is not true. All you are doing is allowing the subconscious mind to come forward, and the subconscious is many times more powerful than the conscious mind. So in effect, you are taking control by going into a hypnotic trance.

Don't worry about having to read the instructions while going through the process the first few times. It will not inhibit you. After a while you will have this method memorized and be able to do it at any time you wish without looking at any instructions.

1. Start by getting comfortable in bed, sitting in a comfortable chair, or lying down where you are safe and comfortable. Once you feel relaxed and at ease, gently close your eyes.
2. Start to tune into your breathing. Inhale for 5 seconds, hold the breath for 3 seconds, and breathe out for 5 seconds. Do this consciously for a while, and the subconscious will soon take over this rhythmic breathing.
3. Focus on a point in your mind. I always recommend 'looking' at the point between your eyebrows, your 'third eye'. This point of focus will become your 'screen'. Notice the color of the screen – typically it is black or orange.
4. Become aware of any random thoughts that come into your head. Acknowledge the thought, then allow it to pass from your mind. If you get hung up on a particular thought that is ok, wait a while and this too will pass.

5. Picture yourself lying on soft green grass in a field. It is a beautiful cloudless day, except for one white fluffy cloud. You are watching this cloud. Now keep watching as it makes its way slowly across the sky. Keep watching until you are no longer interested in the cloud. Keep relaxing and breathing rhythmically.

6. Now see yourself at the top of a staircase that has 10 steps. If you wish, you can visualize the staircase in great detail, noticing a very secure handrail. Now step off onto the first step. Inhale and exhale once per step. As you step down tell yourself to let go of all tension in the body. On the next step give yourself permission to go deeper into a trance state. As you step down allow yourself to go deeper and deeper into a relaxed, trance-like state. On each of the last 3 steps, tell yourself to go deeper:

    Step 8: 'Go 5 times deeper!'
    Step 9: 'Go 10 times deeper!'
    Step 10: 'Go 20 times deeper!'

7. When you reach the bottom see a small hallway with a single closed door. Take a final releasing breath, open the door and step into your subconscious mind.

8. You can either start making suggestions to yourself immediately, or you can wait a while and see if your subconscious has any messages for you.

Making 'Suggestions' to Yourself While in Self-Hypnosis

Suggestions are what your subconscious mind accepts as truths, while in hypnosis. So you want to 'feed' your mind the best kind of information possible to create positive changes in your life. Think of suggestions as the recipe for your mind to follow.

In your very relaxed state you have reached a brainwave state that is low alpha (brainwave states were discussed earlier in the book). In this state, your critical filter is bypassed and you can make beneficial suggestions to your subconscious mind. Over time, constant repetition will imprint these suggestions onto the subconscious mind. In effect, you will have learned to reprogram your subconscious mind using a set of suggestions that you design to fit the change you would like to facilitate. While this might only be for weight loss purposes, you can extend this to include manifestation, self-esteem, success, and health and wealth type of suggestions as well. With each set of suggestions, adding in some positive affirmations as well, is always a good idea.

Here is a list of powerful suggestions and techniques to assist with weight loss. You will resonate with some more than others. Use those that you think are the most powerful:

Imagery – the New You

Create a picture in your mind of the 'perfect you'. See where this picture is. Is it in your mind or somewhere in your body? Notice the detail of the picture; if the picture is in black and white, give it a powerful burst of color; now increase the detail, make it a high-resolution picture. Now enlarge the picture, blow it up to as big as you are comfortable with. Now study this picture, make any changes you require. Now step into this image, becoming the image and BURN this picture into your mind, into your subconscious. This is the new you, and once your subconscious has it imprinted, it will adopt this as the new reality and will move Heaven and Earth to manifest this new reality. As many times a day as possible, keep submitting this image to yourself. In self-hypnosis, admire this picture in your subconscious mind. Notice how it makes you feel when you are looking at it. Observe it as a third party as well as seeing through the eyes of the new you. Notice how other people are admiring you.

Imagery – a Special Event

Perhaps you have an important function or event in the near future, like your best friend's wedding. If so, focus on the day of the event, and you at your goal weight in a stunning outfit. See the people looking at you, and imagine what they are saying about your new weight, and looking stunning in your new outfit. *Feel* that moment, and burn it into your subconscious. Or summer might be approaching, and you need to slim down to fit into the amazing new swimsuit you bought (or are intending to buy). Picture yourself vividly on the beach, looking slim and toned, and see the people watching you admiringly.

Imagery – Future Projection

Project yourself into a day in the future, where you are your perfect weight. Walk through the day, from when you wake in the morning; what you wear; what you eat;

see yourself going to work, etc. until you climb into bed. Lock in this new reality, and burn it into your subconscious many times in a day (see The Color Red for a technique on this).

Imagery – Shopping Spree

At your new goal weight, many of your clothes will no longer fit you. See yourself on a major shopping spree where you excitedly try on and purchase a brand-new wardrobe. See your friend's expressions when they see your new body in your new clothes. *Feel* how amazing you *feel*, and burn that into your subconscious.

Imagery – Virtual Gastric Band Technique

Many people undergo surgery to remove a piece of the stomach, or to staple the stomach. This achieves a smaller stomach so that you get fuller quicker, and cannot eat as much.

The virtual surgery is just as effective: imagine seeing the doctor who consults and explains the process to you. Imagine your surgery is scheduled a week later. Imagine waking up on that day and packing your bag for the hospital. Imagine walking into the hospital, checking in, and signing all of the forms. Imagine lying in your gurney as you are wheeled into the operating room. Imagine blacking out from the anesthesia (and allow yourself to go even deeper at this stage). Now pretend you are outside of your body looking down on the scene, where you observe the surgeon skillfully decreasing the size of your stomach. When you awaken, your stomach is now the size of a tennis ball. Your appetite will now decrease accordingly.

Imagery – The Control Room

At the bottom of the staircase, you used to deepen yourself, instead of a door you now see an elevator. Step into the elevator and this will take you to the control room in your subconscious mind.

Step out of the elevator and now visualize or imagine this control room in your mind. Stand back in awe at this amazing place that controls all your bodily functions. There are, buttons, knobs, levers, and pulleys; digital control boards, with flashing lights; there are pipes leading into and out of the room.

Now find the fat thermostat. See how the fat thermostat is turned up to its maximum level. Now turn the thermostat down to its lowest possible level. You can be inventive with other controls, such as the exercise dial and the metabolism control dial. You can adjust this at any stage. Anytime you wish, you can return to these dials, and reset them.

The control room, is also very good for controlling pain (see two dials, one comfort and the other pain. See how the pain dial is on full volume, now turn it down to the level you desire. See the comfort level is turned down low, and now turn it up to its maximum level).

Eating Habits

Embrace new eating habits. See yourself eating better foods, reducing carbs and sugar, reducing alcohol, and exercising more. Play through various scenarios in your head and see yourself as you are offered processed high-carb foods and you decline, instead opting for healthy, organic alternatives. Many people feel obligated to eat everything on their plate. If you are one of these people ask yourself 'why?'. Typically, it relates to childhood programming where a parent told you to eat everything on your plate.

Identify where these faulty thoughts are coming from, and where they might live in your mindbody. Now change these thoughts. No harm will come from you leaving food on your plate; in fact, much good will come from it. Lose any guilt you may be carrying around with you as it does not serve your highest good.

From this point on, you will eat until you start feeling full. At that point, you will push the plate away. In your mind, picture a row of food shelves like at the supermarket. The 'bad' foods that you like are currently sitting on the eye-level shelf, easy to see and easy to purchase. One by one, move these items to a shelf so high, you cannot reach it. Anything sitting on that shelf is so high, it is difficult to even see, and even more difficult to reach. Now place healthy organic food options on the eye-level shelf. When you think of food, the items on the eye-level shelves jump out and scream your name. These items are what you crave from now on.

Emotional Eating

Search your mindbody for the emotion that causes the over-eating. It might be sadness, or self-protection, or eating as a substitute for love, or something entirely different. Be honest with yourself. Realizing why you are over-eating is halfway to fixing the issue. When you find the reason, accept that it is not serving any beneficial purpose. If it is something like self-protection, for instance, agree with your subconscious mind that this protection is not necessary, that you have nothing to fear, and agree to 'let it go.'

Increase Self-Image, Confidence, Self-Love, Inner-Peace

Often the emotional 'cause' of the overweight status is poor self-image, lack of confidence, or lack of self-love. Say your favorite daily affirmations to yourself (but particularly in self-hypnosis). Increasing your self-image, confidence and self-love will remove the need for food as a substitute. In terms of confidence and motivation, remind yourself of past successes and achievements, and how amazing you will feel when you are at your goal weight.

Metaphors – Heavy Coat

Imagine the excess weight you are carrying is like a heavy coat that you are wearing. Imagine how heavy and laborious it is to carry this coat around with you. Now agree to remove this coat, and allow yourself to *feel* how freeing it *feels* without the heavy coat.

Metaphors – the Bully Inside You

If you desire to look amazing, then what part of your mindbody is forcing you to eat badly, or to overeat, or to do no exercise? In hypnosis, search your mindbody and identify this bully. Eject this bully from your mindbody, never to return.

Metaphors – Client Version 2.0

Perhaps you were once at your goal weight. A time you felt great and were really 'comfortable in your own skin.' Go back to that time and take a copy of your DNA. Now paste that DNA into your body, and watch as the cells rapidly replicate, spreading the 'thin you' DNA into your body.

Other Hypnotic Suggestions for Weight Loss

- Exercise—even walking five minutes every day has a beneficial effect. Suggest to yourself to start easily, and work up to moderate exercise; 'I love my everyday walks'.
- Removing fat—every day our body naturally removes fat through breath, excretion, normal sweat, and exercise sweat. Give your body permission to accelerate this fat removal: to visualize breathing more and to see more fat excreted in every drop of sweat; 'My body is a fine-tuned machine and burns off fat quickly as I

go through my day'.

- Impulses—mind hunger versus real hunger—sometimes we eat when we are bored or anxious, and not when we are hungry. Be mindful of eating only when you are hungry. Sometimes we think we are hungry, but in fact, we are really only thirsty—see yourself drinking more water before you eat. 'I love to drink a big glass of water before every meal'.
- Reduce appetite—food has lots of energy (calories) and the body does not require so many calories. Therefore, minimize the intake of non-necessary calories; 'I am not interested in eating as much food as I was in the past'.
- Mindful eating—life is all about choices, so from this point on be mindful of your choices, be present when you eat food and not distracted by other activities; 'I like to really enjoy and experience my food and focus on it as I eat'.

The Color Red

Imagine yourself, or another person saying this to you: 'You are going to find and discover that the color red is going to be a little brighter, a little sharper to you than ever before, whether it is a taillight, stoplight, stop sign, color of a car or clothing.

It could be as small as nail polish or as large as a billboard. The color red is going to seem sharper and brighter than ever before and each and every time your mind encounters the color red, you can state what will happen.

Such as what emotions will be triggered, that you will have willpower, perseverance, or anything that will help you in the process. For example: 'My desire, determination, motivation, and inner drive to shed any excess weight will become stronger and stronger each and every day. And once I have reached my desired goal, I will easily and with little effort, remain my perfect weight)'

Awakening

If you are lying in bed and your intention for self-hypnosis is to completely relax in order to get to sleep, then obviously no awakening is required. If you are sitting in a chair and performing self-hypnosis during your lunch break, and you now have to go back to work, drive a car, or operate machinery, then obviously you need to come out of hypnosis.

1. Tell your mind the session is over and you wish to be fully awake.
2. Count from zero to five. At five say 'Wide Awake!' So, you say 'One, Two Three, Four, Five, Wide Awake!' You can also 'pump your fists', which means to make a fist, then relax it, then repeat that process a few times using both hands. The right fist stimulates the left side of your brain, and the left fist stimulates the right.
3. Change your position (if sitting—stand; if lying down—sit or stand).

Tips for Self-Hypnosis:

- Sit or lay down somewhere comfortable and get into a state of relaxation.
- Unlike meditation, there is no need to clear your mind, but do focus on the steps.
- Take your time and do not rush the counting steps.
- With countdown scripts, how far you countdown will depend on you and how you feel. There is no magic number. Experiment and go with what feels right for you.
- Pause often. When you pause, focus on your breathing. Your breathing is a hypnotic process.
- Allow yourself to drift and relax.
- Learn to embrace and not fear distractions. Acknowledge them and move on, never try to fight them. Say to yourself that each distraction allows you to go deeper (or relax more).
- I choose to do this in my bed, as it is a safe, relaxed place, and the state of relaxation induced by self-hypnosis aids me in getting to sleep. The Law of Association is in effect here—the bed is associated with relaxation and sleep. The resulting alpha state is what we are trying to obtain, to gain access to the subconscious.
- If you are doing self-hypnosis and the intention is not to fall asleep afterward, then ensure you fully awaken.

- Consider whether you want music, or perhaps white noise. If music is used, consider an auto-stop for when you have fallen asleep (unless you want the recording to carry on playing).

The Mental Bank

From the ages of zero to fourteen our mind is like a sponge, readily absorbing everything we see around us. Based on this information we create a script in our subconscious mind. This script dictates our success parameters for the rest of our lives.

A portion of the population is able to bring about effective changes in their script without using tools such as hypnosis or other methods. The majority of us, however, will require additional tools to assist with this change. The Mental Bank is one of those tools. It is a process that can effectively improve your internal script, so that you will alter what your subconscious believes to be true.

The Mental Bank is a book written by Dr. John Kappas which describes a method of changing your level of homeostasis by a utilizing a daily game-like practice. Between the ages of eight and fourteen, you intensively modeled the behavior of other people and inferred success principles from these people, which formed your life script. The majority of this script was imprinted onto your subconscious mind, and established the limitations you are experiencing today.

The Mental Bank works much like a regular bank, but with the mind. Each night before you go to sleep, you record 'payments' and 'deposits' in the form of activities that you have performed that day. There are certain higher value activities that align with your goals and regular activities.

In the beginning, it is recommended that you take your current income and double it, then divide by working hours to get a standard 'hourly rate.' Payments for tasks/activities you enjoy might be at the 'standard' rate. Payment for activities that are in support of your goals or may be harder to accomplish, might be paid at double-time. You also record what you are grateful for that day. This combination of symbolic wealth/revenue and gratitude creates a virtual income which raises the level of what your subconscious views as its norm...or homeostasis.

The subconscious mind does not know the difference between reality and what is vividly imagined. When we visualize or script something, the information goes into the subconscious mind as if it were real. What we script or visualize ultimately becomes a known to the subconscious mind. So these deposits may as well be in your real bank account.

It is like completing your diary at the end of the day. Doing the Mental Bank process right before you climb into bed is a good idea because your mind starts to slow down at this time and your brainwaves become slower as well. They start to enter an 'alpha' brainwave state (which is just a slower frequency) much the same frequency as the hypnotic state. Therefore, during this window of time in which your subconscious is more receptive, doing this process can have much more profound effects. Your initial dream state (called pre-cognitive dreams) can then absorb these suggestions into your subconscious while you sleep.

You can get a good understanding of the concept of the Mental Bank at **www.mymentalbank.com**. I recommend obtaining the book *The Mental Bank Ledger* by Dr. John Kappas, with a mobile app that is also available to assist you in applying the concept every day.

Law of Attraction

The Law of Attraction was popularized by the Abraham books by Jerry and Esther Hicks, and in later years the concept became more well-known in the mainstream with the release of *The Secret*.

The 'simple' formula:

- Visualization + Enthused Emotion = Manifestation
- Visualization + Inspired Action = Materialization

But like any art/skill, the process of learning it leads to an intuitive 'knowing.' It becomes part of you. By following these guidelines, you will have a blueprint to become a master of the Law of Attraction.

The basic premise of The Law of Attraction is that what

you focus on is attracted into your life. You are supposed to visualize the outcome and believe it to be true. But there is much more to it than that.

When practicing the Law of Attraction and 'summoning,' your desired result, there are several laws which have a strong impact on any Law of Attraction or imagery concept:

- **Law of Reverse Action** – This works on the basis that your mind will respond to a stronger suggestion, if the alternative presented is considerably weaker. It also means that any idea, vision, or concept that resides in your <u>subconscious</u> if it is stronger than reality, will manifest and override a <u>conscious</u> idea, vision or concept. This is why with your conscious mind when you try hard to change your thinking, your life, and your circumstances, often you get little or no result. A good example is when you try to force yourself to go to sleep, and you remain awake for a long time. This is how many people experience the Law of Attraction. Their focus on the fact they are awake, makes them continue to be so. Your subconscious mind is very powerful. When you let your subconscious mind do the heavy lifting, results start to happen.
- **The Law of Repetition** – This law works on the basis that the more we do something, the better at it we become, and the more acceptable it is to us. By repeating your idea, vision or concept as often as you can, it starts to take root. New

neuropathways are being created in the brain, which make a new process into a new habit. This is also linked to the Law of Probability.

- **The Law of Dominance** – The more you believe in your idea, vision or concept, the more real you make it. As in the sayings 'faith can move mountains' and 'if you think you can, or you think you can't you are right'.

- **The Law of Delayed Action** – Some people get disheartened because they do not see instant or rapid materialization of their idea, vision or concept. Trust that the Universe has a grand plan, and that things will happen when they are supposed to. This incorporates letting go, and not being attached to the result.

- **The Law of Association** – Think of some of the things you have materialized in your life. Perhaps as a kid, you pictured the bike you wanted for your birthday, and it materialized. Maybe in little league, you hit that home run. As you think of these instances, feel good about your power of creation. Know that your power works, and it gets stronger with use, like exercising a muscle.

- **Law of Auxiliary Emotion** – The intensity of a suggestion is proportional to the emotion that accompanies it. If the suggestion invoked a weak emotion, it sits but is not firmly anchored in the subconscious. If the suggestion evoked a strong emotion, it is firmly rooted in the subconscious. This is why you need a burst of feel-good energy to 'energize' the idea, vision, or concept and 'burn' it into your subconscious and enhance its strength.

- **Law of Pessimistic Interpretation** – When you have doubts about whether your idea, vision or concept will materialize or not. Remember that humans are naturally pessimistic as a result of a basic survival mechanism. We are constantly looking for possible threats. Go into a higher consciousness, and override this lower level thought process, because most perceived threats are not real threats. Focus on the Law of Association, where you think of times you have successfully manifested other desires.
- **Law of Perception** – If you believe something to be true, it is true for you. Regardless of the reality, you will behave accordingly when you consider something to be true. Keep telling yourself that your vision is true, and it will become so. The mind is a powerful creation tool, which you need to train and exercise.
- **The Law of Belief** – A thought with a known outcome is a fact. You realize what you desire. This is the law that makes any placebo work effectively. The bible mentions this in Mark 11:24: 'Therefore I tell you, whatever you ask in prayer, believe that you have received it, and it will be yours.'
- **Law of Hypnotic Depth (Ewin's Law)** – You do not need to be in a specific brainwave state to practice the law of attraction. However, based on the law of reverse action (your subconscious is stronger than your conscious) and the law of auxiliary emotion (the intensity of a suggestion is

proportional to the emotion that accompanies it), it is best practiced in an alpha state with bursts of gamma energy.

- **The Law of 21** – Most of us have heard that it takes 21 days to form a habit. That is because it takes approximately 21 times to create an automatic trigger mechanism (auto-pilot) that continues to grow stronger with use. A thought will follow an established neural pathway through our mind, but it takes more effort to follow a new one. A new habit is hard to stick to because our mind prefers the easier well-worn neural pathways. Repetition makes the new neuropathways easier to follow. After about twenty-one times, the 'new' routine should become 'habit.' Keep repeating your ideas, vision, and concepts until they become second nature.

- **The Law of Balance/Law of Gratitude** – Life involves balance. For you to 'receive' something, you have to release something, or give something up, or not receive something that was intended for you. Be careful what you ask for, remain in integrity, and always be grateful for what you have. Being grateful ALWAYS attracts more of the same without you having to give something up—because you already have it. You are merely intensifying the quantity.

- **The Law of Homeostasis** – Each of us has a program in our subconscious mind which is our 'script'. This script puts a limit on how successful each of us will be. It enforces our limitations, and sets the ceiling on our successes. But this script can be rewritten, and our subconscious minds can be 'reprogrammed,' using hypnosis, affirmations, gratitude, mindfulness and tools like the Mental Bank. If you do attract success above your pre-programmed limit, there is a good chance you won't retain it. Like exercising your body with weights, you need to exercise your mind's beliefs in order to increase its level of homeostasis.

- **Law of Resistance** – Resistance is fear. For as long as we resist something or somebody in our lives, we are showing fear. Fear is the opposite of attraction. In addition, resistance says that we are not happy with what we have created.

- **The Law of Diminishing Returns** – The harder you try with your conscious mind to design or create manifestations into your life, the less the subconscious will involve itself. If you let your subconscious mind do the heavy lifting, you will require minimal conscious will and effort to create.

- **Law of Probability** – Focus produces results. The more we concentrate on a specific outcome, the more likely that outcome will manifest. Later in the book I prove physically how concentrating on a specific outcome has a greater probability of manifesting that outcome. Add to this the fact that the more you concentrate on something, the more inclined your subconscious is to believe it, and achieve it.

- **The Law of Cycles** – This law applies to the Law of Attraction in that things naturally go 'well' for a while, and things then go 'badly.' Learn to appreciate the ups. Learn to accept the downs. Appreciation will increase the frequency and duration of the ups. A lesson will keep returning until you have learned the lesson; acceptance of the downs will reduce their frequency and duration. What you focus on is what you attract. The Laws of Cycles, Balance and Gratitude are inextricably linked.

The 'Magnetism' Paradox

In describing the Law of Attraction, popular books such as *The Secret* state that 'Everything that exists, has a certain frequency (vibration). Frequencies work magnetically. So, everything that you create, attracts more of the same.'

But this is not technically correct, because in magnetism 'like repels like.' Ergo, if attracting wealth was a result of magnetism, once you had wealth you would then repel wealth. This is not what we want, nor is it how it works. There is, however, the Law of Gratitude, where you resonate with what you have, and so the Universe gives you more of it. And many other laws have an impact on what you are attracting into your life. Rather than a magnet, think in terms of a radio set. Your 'transmitter' sends out messages to the Universe. The Universe sends events and information back to you based on a similar frequency. Your 'receiver' is set to the same frequency as your transmitter. The more powerful your receiver, the more powerful you are in creating and attracting.

You Create Your World

The basic rule of quantum physics is that something can only 'come' into existence **when it is observed**. That means that something can only exist if somebody's mind *first thought it into existence*.

We know our mind is an emitter and receiver of frequencies. What we receive is relative to what we send out. Be conscious of your thoughts, and guard against negative thoughts, emotions and behaviors regarding your body. If you are in the 'right frame of mind' and are sending out the correct frequencies, you will eventually create what you are intending. Fear is a powerful attractor; fear creates focused energy and increases the probability of occurrence. 'You attract your fears' is a valid statement. Fearing the weight attracts it.

Act As If

Thinking about what you want your creation (or your body) to look like is only semi-effective. The most powerful way to create is to act as if it was already there. Act as if you are a billionaire, act as if you are a transcended master, act as if you are a supermodel, etc. Your old creation process of 'think-say-act'' should be turned around—it now becomes 'act-say-think.' For changes to your body, act as if you are that thin person you desire to be. How would they act in any given situation? Your most powerful creation method is by imagining that you already have it!

Focus on What You Really Want

Let's say you want to manifest weight loss. Yet it is not the weight loss you want, it is the freedom, feeling of confidence, choices of clothing, better health and vitality that the loss of the excess weight presents. So instead of focusing on the process, focus on the end result: in this case the confidence, health, etc. that you crave.

Do Not Be Attached to the Outcome

You have heard this multiple time— 'do not be attached to the outcome.' Obviously, this is strange because you desire a particular outcome, and this is why it is a desire. What it really means is this: do not **fear** the outcome, or that the outcome might not manifest. Design an outcome, set your intent, and let it manifest. If it did not manifest, do not be concerned. Merely re-set the intent. Through continuous belief (Laws of Repetition, Perception/Belief, 21, Probability), your subconscious starts to understand and adapt to your design.

Religious/Doctrine Belief

What you perceive as reality, is reality. Some people believe fully in religious texts, such as the Bible. Using elements from these texts is a powerful reinforcement. One example is the Gospel of Mark in the New Testament: 'What things so ever ye desire, when ye pray, believe that ye receive them and ye shall receive them.' Interestingly this statement underlines the Reality Imagery and Law of Perception/Belief discussed above.

Obviously, some people are not religious but reinforcement can be found in many things, from simple memes to deep philosophical statements.

The Power of Gratitude

The power of gratitude is threaded throughout this book. In terms of the Law of Attraction, it is the single most powerful element. For instance, when you state affirmations, consider the following:

- Each and every day my body is in perfect health.
- Each and every day **I AM GRATEFUL** that my body is in perfect health.

The second affirmation is many times more powerful than the first. With any affirmation use present tense ('I am…' as opposed to 'I hope…' or 'I desire…') and 'I am grateful that…' or 'thank you for…'

We see from Dr. Masaru Emoto's work on water crystals, and the beauty of the crystals associated with 'Love and Gratitude' that, when combined, these words are far more powerful than 'Love' or 'Gratitude' on their own. Despite this, 'Gratitude' is one of the most powerful forces in the world. When applying the law of attraction, know that gratitude is a powerful amplifier.

Gratitude is an emotion expressing appreciation for what one has—as opposed to an emphasis on what one wants. When you express gratitude for what you have, the Universe reacts and manifests more of what you are grateful for.

I once attended a seminar by Dr. John Demartini, and he related the following story: Demartini had a billionaire friend who, when asked how he became a billionaire, replied: 'Every night I run through all the events of the day, giving gratitude for everything. In the beginning, it took a long time, but now it takes me five minutes every evening.' In effect, this billionaire concentrates hard for five minutes a day. The good vibrations his gratitude creates attract the experiences and events that contribute to his manifesting the life of a billionaire.

So, ask yourself—do you want to toil endlessly for eight or more hours, every day, to eke out a living, or does it make sense to take a short time during the day to do a gratitude meditation?

There are several ways to improve your life script, to reprogram it. One of the ways is constant gratitude. The Law of Attraction suggests that thoughts are energy. Gratitude is a thought energized with a strong amplifying emotion. Many scientific studies show that we can deliberately embody a culture of gratitude and appreciation to increase our overall well-being and happiness.

Remember:

A deep state of gratitude is a combination of blessings and euphoria—giving blessings for your positive state combined with a sense of euphoria because of your positive state. Simply put, gratitude is the most powerful method of manifesting your intentions and weight loss is deeply connected to your mindbody. Therefore, gratitude for your body, your mind's connection to it, the proper functioning and metabolism, etc. are essential to manifesting a successful outcome.

Chapter 8: Metabolism and the Gut Biome

Training your mind is the most important aspect of your weight loss strategy. Thereafter you can focus on the mechanics, such as metabolism, gut flora, and nutrition. Educating yourself on how the body works and metabolizes the food you put into it is essential in taking control of your health and physique.

Fat Cells

The body does not create new fat cells. Where fat needs to be stored, the body inserts it into existing fat cells. So our fat cells have the ability to become larger as we deposit more into them. The amount of fat successfully processed by the body is dependent on your metabolism and gut-biome (or gut flora). The more efficient these two are, the less chance of fat being deposited. So how can we make them more efficient?

Avoid Prolonged Sitting

Our bodies are not designed to be sedentary. The average person spends more time sitting (office, commuting, or in front of the TV or computer) in a day than they do sleeping. Prolonged sitting negatively impacts our metabolism—and slows it down to about one calorie per minute. This is why long-distance truck drivers struggle with obesity. Lymph vessels remove toxins from our body and they require rhythmic contraction of the muscles in the legs to perform properly. If we are not moving, our lymphatic system is not functioning correctly. If toxins are not removed they end up in stored fat, which makes the fat 'untouchable.'

The body will not burn this fat because it is protecting against the release of toxins into the body. Sitting causes muscles to atrophy. Muscle uses more calories, therefore less muscle = fewer calories burned.

Breathing Exercises

Fat is removed from the body in three ways: excretion (urine/feces), secretion (perspiration) and respiration (breathing). Of the three, breathing is the most effective fat removal process.

A recent study found that, when 10 pounds of fat was oxidized by the body, 8.4 pounds of this fat was converted and excreted as carbon dioxide (CO_2) via the lungs, and 1.6 pounds became water (H_2O), excreted via sweat and/or urine.

So 84% of fat is removed from the body by breathing. Interestingly, in order for 10 pounds of human fat to be oxidized, the researchers calculated that 29 pounds of oxygen must be inhaled. So, it turns out that deep breathing is one of the most effective tools in weight loss.

Consumption of oxygen is proportional to our metabolic rate: increased cellular activity burns more fuel and demands more oxygen. Breathing deeply has a reciprocal effect—it raises the metabolism of your cells. So, breathe deeply people!

Importance of the Digestive System

A lot of people do not understand the impact of the digestive system on overall health, and particularly weight. Food is either a medicine, a neutral, or a toxin. You should be mindful of what and when you eat. Studies done on the gut microbiome have identified 'fat' and 'skinny' bacteria. In essence, eating fiber produces beneficial bacteria: the bacteria thrive on the fiber, and the fiber seems to spawn the healthy bacteria. Large quantities of fiber-related bacteria are found in lean people, whereas very few in obese people. Bottom line: Eat more fiber.

Water, and Chewing

Drinking a glass of water thirty minutes before a meal leads to neuro signals indicating the stomach is partially full, and/or has received nutrients recently. The net effect is you will eat less during the meal, and fewer calories are taken in. Food should be chewed for an abnormally long time. This aids digestion, but also gives the stomach time to send the 'partially-full' signal.

The Importance of Serotonin

A high carb intake (e.g., sugar, bread, cereals, refined flours, etc.) creates a release of insulin in the body. Insulin removes all amino acids (except tryptophan) by pushing them into muscles. Tryptophan is a precursor for serotonin. Serotonin makes us feel good. As insulin has removed all the other amino acids, tryptophan now easily finds available receptors in the brain, which leads to increased serotonin in the body.

high sugar = high insulin = more serotonin.

Interestingly, exercise has the same effect, which is part of the reason we feel so good afterwards.

The main reason for an addiction to bread, pastries, and candy is because of the serotonin ''rush' they deliver to our body. Over time we become tolerant to this unbalanced release of serotonin. We become desensitized and, like any drug, we then need more of it, and more often, to achieve the same 'high.'

If we consider that symptoms of serotonin deficiency are low self-esteem, insomnia, phobias, panic attacks, eating disorders, depression, anger, anxiety, shyness, and obsessive behaviors—as well as cravings for sweets and chocolates, cravings for sweets at night, and binge eating—then we realize just how important serotonin is, especially in regard to weight management.

Alcoholics are addicted to the sugar in alcohol, and the neurohormones released. Carboholics are addicted to the serotonin rush released by the sugars in the carbohydrates. So how can we boost our serotonin production without eating more sugar? The most important part of our immune system is in the gut. The healthier our gastrointestinal system, the healthier our immune system.

The healthier our immune system, the more serotonin we produce. Improving our gut health and boosting serotonin requires attention to:

- Diet
- Exercise
- Sleep
- Exposure to sunlight
- Minimizing stress levels
- Social interaction, particularly intimacy
- Supplements, like 5-HTP and tryptophan. Be careful here—sometimes the body becomes reliant on a supplement and stops making its own.

Serotonin thrives in the right environment and sufficient B vitamins, calcium, magnesium, and vitamin D3, are also required to make it. Exercising outside on a sunny day, and then ingesting an organic, high-fat, grass-fed yogurt, would be an example of making choices that maximize serotonin production. Bear in mind that neurochemicals need to be released in balanced amounts, or we become desensitized to them, and need more of them to achieve the same reward effect.

Eating Time Theories

Theories abound regarding schedule and regularity of eating meals. Nutritionists recommend everything from fasting, limiting to one meal per day, three meals and six snacks per day, not eating before a certain time, not eating after a certain time, etc. Because there are so many opposing theories, it is difficult to know what is correct. Add to that, that all people are different.

Melatonin helps sleep which helps the diet process, BUT melatonin binds to receptors on pancreatic cells to suppress insulin secretion. This occurs in order to keep blood glucose levels steady during the overnight fast. So melatonin acts to suspend the digestive process. This is why late-night eating is not a good idea.

Healthy Vagus Nerve

The vagus nerve is the superhighway connecting our brain, to our gut, and to most areas of our body. It has a delicate electric signaling structure, which includes letting the brain know the stomach is full, the release of gut hormones to the brain, etc. When our vagus nerve is not functioning properly, our whole digestive process will not function properly. One of the main reasons you might be overweight is a malfunctioning vagus nerve. I cannot cover the vagus nerve within the scope of this book, but I encourage you to read up on it.

Feeling Full

If not feeling full is the reason you carry on eating, then, along with protein, increase your intake of healthy fats, such as nuts, coconut oil, avocado, olive and nut oils, and fatty fish.

Toxins in Our Fat

Body fat that contains toxins cannot be broken down and eliminated without removing the toxins first. We encounter toxins in our everyday life. These are taken into the body through poor food, preservatives, chemicals, heavy metals, and pesticides. There are two types of toxins: water- or fat-soluble. The body easily disposes of the water-soluble types. The problem is the fat-soluble toxin: the liver bears the burden of converting them into water-soluble ones for easy disposal.

In a healthy body, with minimal toxins, the liver can perform its job. However, we generally ingest way more toxins than we can safely digest—the liver is overworked, health issues debilitate the system, and modern-day stress can essentially bring this process to a halt. In this non-healthy situation, the body stores the fat-soluble toxins in body fat, particularly around the abdominal area.

Since a primary role of your body + mind + subconscious mind is self-preservation, fat containing toxin is 'separated' from the body. The body refuses to burn this fat for fuel because of the resulting unwanted release of fat-soluble toxins into it. Releasing these toxins would poison the body, and stress all the systems. So, the body 'locks-away' this toxic fat, leaving you with areas of stubborn fat, normally around the abdominal area. If this fat is to be removed, the toxins have to be dealt with first. Only then will the body consider breaking it down.

Detoxification can be achieved through healthy eating (preferably organic), with large amounts of green leafy vegetables (they have a chelating effect, helping remove heavy metals from the body), vitamins and supplements, generous amounts of pure, filtered, preferably alkaline water (not tap water), sleep, rest, mindfulness and meditation.

Once the body has been detoxified, toxins stored in fat will start to be removed. In other words, carry on the detoxification until you see the stubborn fat start to disappear. As the toxins in this fat are removed, you should see the fat start to melt away.

Metabolism

When we diet, our metabolism slows down. This is obviously self-defeating and the opposite of what we desire. So, the key is to maintain a healthy diet (organic, non-GMO, 75% alkaline foods, plenty of fiber, etc.), but not reduce the amount we eat. The key is to increase our metabolism, and we do this in four ways:

1. Exercise: get that body moving, even if it is only 10 minutes a day. Avoid sitting. When we sit, we slow our metabolism down to 1 calorie per minute.
2. Consistent Eating Pattern: when you 'go on a diet' your body knows you have restricted the calories. Your subconscious' primary role is survival, so it slows down the rate at which you burn calories. This is why diets are counter-productive. And very painful. Never deprive yourself with a diet again. Bear in mind this

does not suggest you should overeat.

3. Breathing: your breathing is a signal of your metabolism. A fire needs oxygen – if you are burning calories at a high rate, your breathing will require more oxygen, more often. The converse is also true – if you develop a rhythmic deep breathing habit, your metabolism will increase. There are many resources and techniques available online to improve your breathing. Breathing is also the most effective way of removing the end result of fat burning (mostly carbon dioxide).

4. Gut biome: your metabolism is linked to your gut biome. What you eat dictates the nature of the digestive bacteria in your gut, and the quantity and quality of enzymes you produce. Eat plenty of fiber and organic foods. Increase vegetable intake and reduce simple carbs, especially 'white' foods. See next chapter for nutrition to improve the gut biome.

Chapter 9: Nutrition

Nutrition

Quality nutrition is very important. No amount of hypnotherapy or reprogramming will help if you are bingeing daily on a dozen donuts:

- **Glucose Sensitivity** – if this is a possible factor, test and/or see your doctor.
- **Low-Carb / High-Fat Diet** – the old high carb diet was a fallacy. One only has to look at how obese America has become to realize it does not work. An effective diet is low carb and high (healthy) fats. Research the Banting diet, or current authors like Jorge Cruise's *The 100 Diet* and David Zinczenko's *Zero Belly Diet*.
- **Healthy Fats** – The villain becomes the hero. For so many years fat was the enemy, but numerous studies (and common sense) now reveal how much our bodies require these fats. Butter (preferably grass-fed) is not only healthy for you, but margarine which was marketed as a healthy alternative is actually a toxic plastic that should not be commercially available. Cook freely with coconut oil, and butter, and use olive oil in salads (oils like olive oil have a low flashpoint, so it is best not to heat them). Coconut oil has been linked to a multitude of benefits including improved weight loss.
- **Xylitol** – you may or may not have heard of this sugar substitute. It is a natural substance made from the bark of a birch tree. Our bodies produce

up to fifteen grams of xylitol daily as part of the normal metabolic process. Sugar has a glycemic index of 100, whereas Xylitol has a glycemic index of 7. It has lower carbs than sugar, tastes the same and is beneficial for your teeth, even repairing cavities. Stevia is another good option.

- **Mindful Eating** – our modern lifestyle has lead us to embrace fast food and eating on the run. We rarely have time to sit, breathe correctly, savor our food, and chew our it thoroughly, and have time to focus on the food and give gratitude for it. Meals should become ritualized in order to remove added stress elements from our lives.

- **Food Ledger** – Writing down what you eat makes you more aware of how much you are consuming and studies show it reduces the amount of food consumed. An added boost to this tool is to log the caloric content as well. You can look up food's calorie content (a good database is available at **http://ndb.nal.usda.gov/**). Seeing how many calories you are ingesting, brings this information into your conscious awareness, so that you to slow down your food intake, and make healthier choices.

- **Customized Nutrition Plan** – if you have a planned set of meals, you are less likely to 'grab something from the fridge' or head out for fast food. Planning ahead means you can shop and have all the necessary ingredients, or premade smartly-portioned healthy meals in the cupboard and fridge. Meal preparation can be done in the evening for the following day.

- **Hydration** – water is very important to health and weight loss. Choosing water means you are not choosing an alternative with calorie-laden alternatives and water is necessary to flush toxins and hydrate cells. You also burn calories to digest it, and it improves removal systems which help remove fat. In a study, participants who drank 500 ml of water thirty minutes before a meal, lost approximately ten more pounds than those who did not drink water. Our liver removes toxins, and those toxins it cannot remove are stored in fatty tissue. The liver needs extra water to 'flush' these toxins before fatty tissue can be eliminated from the system.

- **Protein as a Snack** – when you have a need for a snack, protein is a good choice — such as a bag of almonds or a slice of cheese. It slows down the absorption of carbohydrates, which helps to avoid blood sugar spikes.

- **Importance of Organic Foods** – organic food is like medicine for our bodies. Other food—particularly alcohol and sugar, but also preservatives, chemicals, pesticides, etc., add toxins to our body. These toxins are stored in our fat, which becomes difficult to break down and remove. Organic food has minimal toxins, and helps to remove the toxins from our body. Avoid GMO (Genetically Modified Organisms) and heavily-processed foods, preservatives, and MSG. MSG is an excitotoxin which is a type of chemical (usually amino acids) that overstimulate neuron receptors, so they fire impulses too rapidly that they become exhausted.

- **Dangers of Sugar** – sugar and fructose (the type of sugar found in fruit) trick the body into creating dopamine. Thus, we become addicted to that dopamine release, which creates an addiction to sugar. Fructose also tricks the body into gaining weight by fooling the metabolism (it turns off the appetite-control system). Fructose does not appropriately stimulate insulin, which in turn does not suppress ghrelin (the 'hunger hormone') and doesn't stimulate leptin (the 'satiety hormone'), which together result in our eating more, and developing insulin resistance. One of the main reasons for America's obesity epidemic is the widespread use of high fructose corn syrup which now pervades our food supply.
- **Dangers of Artificial Sweeteners** – most artificial sweeteners have been linked to kidney failure, coronary disease, nerve damage, digestive malfunction, and insulin resistance. Much of society thinks that because it is approved by the FDA, and freely available, it must be safe. And because of the hype around 'sugar-free,' that it must be healthier to consume than sugar. This is not true. Studies indicate that diet-soda is a major contributor to our obesity epidemic. Artificial sweeteners also increase the urinary excretion of calcium, leading to weakened bones.
- **Dangers of Soda** – one can of soda contains more than the entire recommended daily amount of sugar (via high fructose corn syrup). It creates an insulin spike and your body converts this sugar to

fat. A normal can of soda can contain thirteen teaspoons of sugar. In a typical person, this would induce a vomit response, so the manufacturers add phosphoric acid to dilute the sugar effect. It acts as a diuretic and removes calcium and other minerals from your body. You need zinc, calcium, and magnesium reserves to process the phosphoric acid. This weakens your immune system, leads to calcification of joints, and increases inflammation, particularly arthritis. Diet soda is far worse; a can of diet soda may contain thirteen packets of aspartame. The liver requires one week to process this toxin, which creates poisonous formaldehyde as a by-product.

- **Metabolism** – eat three regular-sized meals, and consume plenty of snacks. On a normal diet your body thinks it is being starved, it slows down the metabolic process as a survival mechanism. The reverse is true—when you continually feed your body the survival mechanism stops and your metabolism increases. A good indicator of faster metabolism is that more oxygen is consumed, and breathing is deeper.

- **Thyroid Regulation** – the thyroid is responsible for hormone regulation, and many of these hormones affect weight loss. Increase iodine intake, especially if you are 'O' blood type.

- **Treats** – you are not a robot and should not deprive yourself from enjoying the occasional treat. This should be encouraged, perhaps as a reward system. When you deviate from the diet it should be done without guilt or shame. Guilt and shame have too many calories!

- **Magnesium** – most overweight people have a magnesium deficiency. Magnesium helps insulin balance and protein utilization and is needed to balance calcium. Magnesium inhibits cortisol (cortisol Is a chemical released in the body that among other negative effects, exacerbates weight gain). The following foods are high in magnesium: nuts, green leafy veggies, whole grains, dairy, and apricots.
- **Aloe Vera** – increases metabolism, stimulates collagen (collagen protein burns calories), and is a natural laxative which helps detoxify the body, and slow sugar absorption.
- **Lectin** – foods high in lectin (soy, potatoes, grains) can be toxic for certain people. In addition, too much lectin interferes with the gut, repair of epithelial cells and causes **leptin** resistance, which is a marker of obese people.
- **Lemons** – polyphenols in lemons, aid in weight loss, boost metabolism, and boost sensitivity to insulin.

Alkaline/Acidity in The Body

Our body is mostly water, and water has a neutral to slightly alkaline pH level. When it is too acidic, it compensates by storing acidic foods as fat. The fewer acidic foods we eat, the less can be stored as fat. As a general rule, 75% of food should be alkaline, 25% acidic.

See the pH levels of foods at:
http://www.energiseforlife.com/us/free-alkaline-food-chart.

The main alkalizing minerals are calcium, iron, magnesium, potassium, and sodium. Foods high in these minerals are considered alkaline-forming food. Most foods have both acid and alkaline minerals in them. If acidic minerals are greater in concentration, that food is considered acidic and vice versa. Saliva contains alkalizing enzymes such as amylase. If you chew food enough, amylase gets the opportunity to help reduce the acidity of the food. Eating quickly, and 'gulping' down liquid, like soda and fruit juice means these enter your stomach in a highly acidic state. When we eat acidic food, our body borrows alkaline from organs and bones—this has the effect of acidifying your body, especially the organs. In science pH stands for 'potential Hydrogen'—for health and weight loss, I want you to think of it as 'perfect Health'. An optimum level for your body is 7.36pH.

Weight Loss and Hormones*

A healthy sleep pattern, sufficient protein intake, and lower carbohydrate intake are all important for proper hormone functioning. Too much or too little of the following hormones can affect weight loss positively or negatively.

These include:

- **Ghrelin:** which tells our body when we are

hungry, and when we are full

- **Leptin:** is another hormone that regulates cravings
- **Cholecystokinin:** stimulates the digestion of fat and protein
- **Insulin:** regulates fat storage
- **Irisin:** is released by muscle tissue, particularly during and after exercise and aids weight loss. Irisin converts white fat to brown fat.

Some obesity markers include:

- High Estrogen,
- Low Testosterone
- Low DHEA (a hormone of the adrenal glands)
- High Insulin
- High Cortisol

Abdominal Fat

Abdominal fat in men increases the conversion of testosterone into estrogen, which leads to increased abdominal fat—this is a vicious cycle. Protein, zinc, and exercise all help a male create testosterone. Abdominal obesity is linked to reduced growth hormone. Growth hormone is released during deep sleep (melatonin induces this) and while we exercise. If hormones are an indicated factor in your weight issue, you may wish to consult a hormone replacement therapist.

Obesity Trend Linked to FDA Recommended Diet

Since the government-approved guidelines were introduced and recommended in the 1970s, and particularly the guideline from 1984, obesity levels increased and continue to spike (see the following chart). The government has a history of making poor nutritional and dietary recommendations.

One reason is the funding they get from special interest groups. Sugar, GMO, grain—they all have powerful organizations with vested interests, translating into campaign contributions that sway government decisions. My point here is not political—it is up to each of us to listen to our inner voice when making decisions on food and medicine.

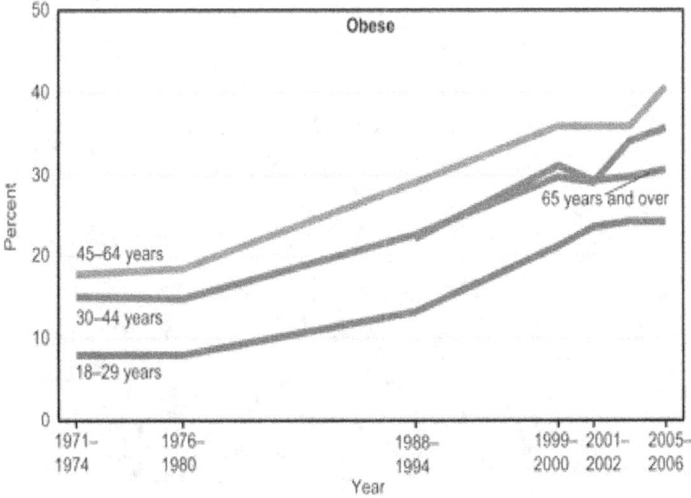

*Chart courtesy of US National Center for Health Statistics

Just because the government recommends it, does not make it the right choice.

The Old Food Pyramid Versus the New Pyramid

Since the early '70s, the Food and Drug Administration recommended a diet (aptly named S.A.D.) high in cereals, grains, and carbohydrates, moderate in protein and low in fats.

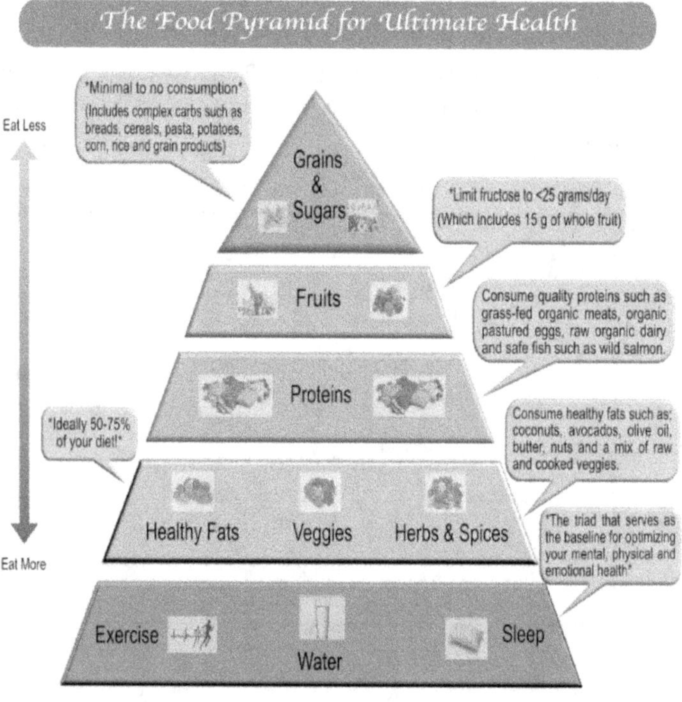

Synthetic products like margarine were preferred to their 'fat-rich' cousin, butter. Many things are wrong with the recommendations, one of which is that our body converts carbohydrates into sugar and 'good' fats are lumped in with 'bad' fats.

The world is now noticing how necessary fats are in a diet and that natural, preferably organic, products like grass-fed butter are far healthier for you than 'Frankenfoods' like margarine and vegetable oil..

The old recommended diet led to an obesity epidemic, with accompanying illnesses and poor health conditions. People have finally woken up and are embracing diets low in carbs, with minimal sugar, and high in healthy fats. This diagram outlines an optimal diet

There were many aspects of the old government recommended diet that were wrong, and actually encouraged obesity. Some foods were promoted that should not be - corn, dairy, sugar – and some foods like butter and coffee were demonized. Coffee alone provides the majority of Americans with the bulk of their antioxidant intake.

Another example is selenium; the S.A.D. diet reduced intake of meat, eggs, and nuts. Your thyroid is the main regulator of your metabolism and needs selenium to function properly. The best sources of selenium are meat, eggs and nuts.

Foods, Herbs, Hormones, and Supplements that Aid Weight loss

- **Protein:** Boosts metabolism; burns more calories to digest than taken in; is not converted to sugar (and then stored as fat) like carbohydrates; and helps build muscle, which burns more calories than fat.
- **Apple Cider Vinegar:** Stimulates digestion, improves metabolism, regulates blood sugar, and the pectin in ACV makes you feel full.
- **B-Vitamins:** In general, B vitamins keep stress under control, and help to burn fat by augmenting protein digestion. B12 especially helps to metabolize fat. The following foods are high in B Vitamins: dark green leafy veggies, poultry, beef, fish, shellfish and eggs and whole grains.
- **Vitamin C:** Inflammation can promote weight gain (some inflammation affects fat storage—we call this 'fatflammation') and Vitamin C helps reduce inflammation. It also aids metabolism. The following foods are high in vitamin C: dark green leafy veggies, red bell peppers, strawberries, kiwi and citrus fruits.
- **Vitamin D3:** People with low vitamin D levels tend to gain weight more easily and quickly than those with high levels. Vitamin D3 helps reduce inflammation (fatflammation). The best form of vitamin D3 is sunlight, which allows the body to produce its own vitamin D, as well as linked beneficial chemicals (like nitric-oxide). The

following foods are high in vitamin D: fish, eggs, and mushrooms.

- **Magnesium:** Most overweight people have a magnesium deficiency. Magnesium helps insulin balance and protein utilization and is needed to balance calcium. Magnesium inhibits cortisol (cortisol exacerbates weight gain). The following foods are high in magnesium: green leafy veggies, whole grains, dairy, and apricots.

- **Omega-3 fats:** These are beneficial to weight loss, and reduce inflammation (fatflammation). People who include this in their diet lose more weight. The following foods are high in omega-3 fats: fatty sea fish (wild-caught), shrimp, DHA-enriched eggs, grass-fed beef, walnuts, chia seeds, and algae-derived docosahexaenoic acid (DHA).

- **Selenium:** Our thyroid governs our metabolism. Selenium aids the thyroid. The following foods are high in selenium: beef, poultry, fish, eggs, and Brazil nuts.

- **Fiber:** Decreases ghrelin, the appetite hormone. Slows release of sugars into the bloodstream, which helps to keep blood sugar levels steady. Keeps us feeling fuller. Promotes regular bowel movements. The following foods are high in fiber: most veggies, avocado, beans/legumes, whole grains, chia seeds, flax seeds, and nuts.

- **Calcium:** Calcium regulates fat storage and usage, improves thermogenesis (the process of energy production in the body caused by the metabolizing of food consumed), targets belly fat, and keeps weight off. Sufficient calcium in the body deters appetite, as insufficient calcium prompts the body to ask for food. The following foods are high in calcium: sesame seeds, chia seeds, dark leafy greens, oranges, quinoa, blackstrap molasses (but beware sugar content), beans, broccoli, dried fruit, nuts, and dried herbs.

- **Chromium:** Regulates blood sugar, curbs cravings for carbs, and improves insulin resistance. The following foods are high in chromium: processed meats, whole-grain products, high-bran cereals, green beans, broccoli, nuts, and egg yolk. Simple sugars cause excretion of chromium.

- **Leptin:** Leptin signals the brain that we are full, and increases metabolic function. Our body makes leptin (in adipose tissue) and cannot absorb it from food sources. The secret lies in regulating our own leptin (similar to insulin regulation), by eating healthy foods, minimizing simple carbs, eliminating white foods (sugar, flour, rice, potatoes), and eliminating sweeteners. Eat protein (especially for breakfast), omega-3s, dark leafy veggies, and increase zinc intake.

- **Green Tea:** Increases fat burn, reduces inflammation (fatflammation), increases norepinephrine.

- **Norepinephrine:** People with a norepinephrine deficiency are never full and always crave starchy foods. How our body makes norepinephrine: phenylalanine becomes tyrosine, which becomes dopamine which becomes norepinephrine. Foods high in phenylalanine include meat, fish, and some dairy like cottage cheese. Foods high in tyrosine include meat and dairy as well as bananas and seaweed.

- **Serotonin:** Lack of serotonin causes weight gain. Serotonin suppresses appetite. Lack of serotonin increases cravings and presence of serotonin reduces cravings. Ironically, glucose produces tryptophan which is the building block for serotonin. Protein also has tryptophan, but our body does not absorb this well because the protein fights for the same receptors (and tryptophan is 'lazy' so cannot find available receptors).
- **Caffeine:** suppresses appetite and increases fat burn. Thermogenic.
- **Green Coffee Bean:** chlorogenic acid controls sugar and increases fat burn.
- **Raspberry Ketones (rheosmin):** increases fat burn
- **Garcinia Cambogia:** suppresses appetite and speeds up metabolism.
- **Frauenmantle Leaf Extract:** suppresses appetite and speeds up metabolism.
- **Wild Olive Leaf:** suppresses appetite and speeds up metabolism.
- **Cormino Seed Extract:** suppresses appetite and speeds up metabolism.
- **Horsemint Leaf Extract:** suppresses appetite and speeds up metabolism.
- **Ginseng:** speeds metabolism and improves insulin sensitivity.
- **Cayenne Pepper:** shrinks fat, lowers blood fat, thermogenic, increases metabolism.
- **Cinnamon:** blood sugar regulator, lowers

appetite, speeds metabolism.

- **Black Pepper:** prevents formation of new fat cells, fat burner when combined with capsaicin.
- **Mustard:** greatly speeds metabolism.
- **Turmeric/Curcumin:** reduces formation of fat tissue, improves insulin resistance, and reduces inflammation (fatflammation).
- **Ginger:** anti-inflammatory (fatflammatory), thermogenic, speeds metabolism, appetite suppressant.
- **Cardamom:** thermogenic, boosts fat burn.
- **Cumin:** aids digestion and improves glycemic control.
- **Hoodia:** I do not recommend hoodia, but there is a lot of hype regarding this (and that is why I include it here). At best, it is an appetite suppressant.
- **Rhodiola:** activates lipase, accelerates breakdown of fat stored in adipose tissue.
- **Fenugreek:** contains a free amino acid (4-hydroxyisoleucine) which manages insulin-promotion and glucose regulation.
- **Yerba Maté:** suppresses appetite and boosts metabolism.
- **Avocado:** rich in cancer-fighting lipids, fiber, vitamins and minerals. The good fats in avocados force out the bad fats.
- **Olives:** rich in cancer-fighting phytonutrients and compounds. Olives are low in carbs and contain fat-fighting compounds.
- **Guayusa:** boosts metabolism and balances blood.

Note: many other foods/herbs/supplements that claim to aid weight loss have been legally banned. One of these is epinephrine because of toxicity to the cardiovascular system.

Food Combinations

Some combinations of food have a positive effect—such that the whole is more than the sum of its parts. One example is Golden Milk, a combination of coconut milk and turmeric, which stimulates the thyroid gland, our metabolism control. Another example is grapefruit juice mixed with olive oil, which stimulates bile, breaks down toxins and fatty deposits in the liver. Once the liver is healthy, it focuses on metabolizing fat stores.

Coconut Oil

Coconut oil is extremely beneficial for weight loss. It has many medium-chain saturated fatty acids which do not get stored in adipose tissue (mostly monounsaturated fats get stored there). It reduces appetite, is thermogenic and boosts metabolism. Our body stores toxins in fatty tissue, and the fat cannot be broken down until the toxins have been removed. Coconut oil assists in this detoxification.

White is Not Right

'White' foods tend to be simple sugars and acidic in nature. Avoid 'white' foods—such as sugar, artificial sugar, rice, flour, pasta, table salt, white wine and even white vinegar—as much as possible. All have a pH of 5.5 or lower which means they are very acidic. Potatoes and milk are only slightly better. In its natural form, salt does not have a pH balance, but additives to table salt make it toxic. Pure salt, like Himalayan, and to a lesser extent sea salt, are alkaline. The body stores acidic food that cannot be processed immediately as fat.

Part of the reason that these 'white' foods are not good for weight loss is that they contribute to leptin sensitivity. Leptin resistance is a marker of obese people. Leptin is a hormone in the body that controls hunger and feelings of satiety. Leptin is secreted by adipose (fat) tissue, so the more overweight a person is, typically, the higher his leptin levels. Ordinarily this would be a good thing, however, the fat works in a way which confuses and negates leptin signals to the brain.

The more 'easily digestible' a food is, the more fattening it is because it causes insulin to spike. Starches, refined flour, and liquid carbohydrates are prime suspects in this regard. This causes a downward spiral where the body starts to become insulin resistant, which ultimately leads to weight gain.

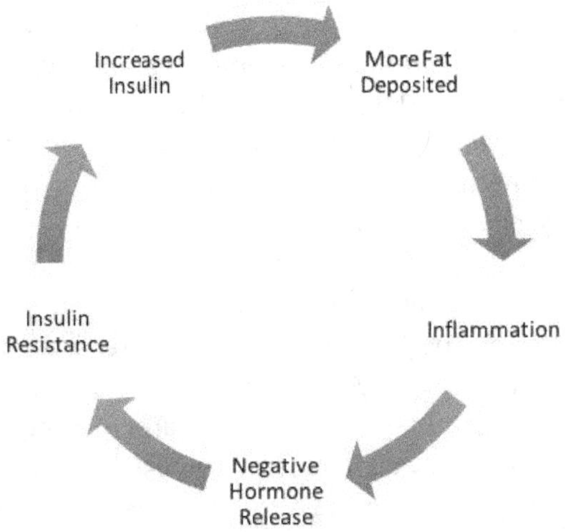

Sugar in particular should be eliminated from the diet:

- Sugar makes us crave more sugar—it hijacks the brain's reward pathway and makes 'users' dependent, creating a neurochemical addiction to sugar.
- Sugar affects our gut biome in a negative way.
- Sugar has a negative effect on the production of insulin. Insulin regulates fat storage; therefore, sugar has a direct impact on fat storing.
- Sugar spikes dopamine release, which desensitizes us to dopamine. This leads to a lowered reward from other 'pleasurable' activities. We then need more 'bad stuff' (e.g., pastries) to give us the same high.

Be Prepared. Emergency Food Packs . . .

The reasons we do not stick to a planned dietary schedule are: availability, time to make and convenience. When we get home after a long day and think about food, two things pop into our mind: convenience and availability. If there is something pre-made in the fridge, then that is our automatic choice. We can learn from this:

- Plan weekly meals in advance.
- List all the ingredients we require to stick to our healthy plan. Make sure we have a surplus of the ingredients. If one or two are missing, we will more easily deviate from the planned meal.
- Pre-prepare as much of the meal as reasonably possible. This cuts down on preparation time and helps resist temptation when it comes to choosing.
- Reward for sticking to the plan. May I suggest a reward being an occasional glass of wine or a tequila? The wine and tequila have alleged slimming properties, while the wine also has a health benefit. Perhaps the glass of wine enjoyed with dinner is the motivation for sticking to the meal schedule. Raw dark chocolate (one of the best sources of antioxidants) is another acceptable sin.
- Make 'emergency packs.' These could be prepared on the weekend for use on workdays. They might consist of almonds, a healthy snack bar, other types of nuts, seeds, nut butters, coconut oil, wild-caught salmon, free-range chicken or turkey, berries, etc. If these are to be lunch packs, I suggest putting them in Ziploc bags

in the fridge, one for each day to grab as you set off for work.

Meds Do Not Help Weight loss

If you are taking medication you should be aware that many lead to weight gain, particularly those used to treat schizophrenia, bipolar disorders, depression, epilepsy, diabetes, blood pressure and migraines.

One reason for this is that they block 'normal' body functions, which means exactly that—the body cannot function normally. This is the reason we have to take med 'A' to overcome the side effects of med 'B,' to overcome the side effects of med 'C,' etc. Another reason meds do not aid weight loss is because they generally have an acidic pH.

Another danger of modern meds is the lack of awareness. Take cholesterol for instance – this has been painted as a dangerous demon to be minimized and controlled. Only now is medical science finding that cholesterol is not a demon at all in terms of weight loss and heart health. In fact, cholesterol is vital for weight loss: a fat molecule is large, too large for the body to handle. The liver and gall bladder produce bile to break up these large fat molecules into smaller molecules, so that they can be processed, digested or removed from the body. To create this bile, the body needs cholesterol. One of the evils of the low-fat diet was that less bile is produced, leading to larger fat storage.

Because modern medicine and its 'findings' are often driven and funded by the interests of Big Pharma or other entities who stand to benefit financially from a study's findings, I highly recommend do your own research. Look at studies and claims more in depth, such as finding out who they are conducted and funded by, etc. Don't accept all that is touted as fact.

Glucose Sensitivity/Diabesity

Many people are either pre-diabetic, diabetic, or have glucose sensitivity.

If you are sensitive to glucose there is a likelihood that you will become pre-diabetic, hyperglycemic, or hypoglycemic. If so, you need to pay special attention to what you eat, and when you eat it. Exercise is highly beneficial in regulating blood sugar disorders.

If you believe you are glucose sensitive, there is a questionnaire in the Appendix that you can complete. If you believe you have glucose sensitivity, consult a doctor or specialist for help.

Chapter 10: The Importance of Exercise

Muscles and organs use energy. This energy usage leads to your body 'burning calories'. If your body does not have enough calories from food, it turns to stored resources – the fat on your body. Body fat is the opposite. Fat uses minimal energy, and actively produces hormones which negate the weight loss process. Simply put, the fatter you are, the fatter you will become. Conversely, the fitter you are, the faster your body burns calories.

Muscles and organs are 'MATs': Metabolically Active Tissue. Fat is not MAT, it is a HAT: Hormonally Active Tissue. Sadly, these hormones work against you, such as ghrelin which tells you to eat more. Fat also interferes with body signaling, such as leptin sensitivity.

So, the body is a see-saw: there is a tipping point where you are 'metabolically positive' (you are burning more calories than you ingest) or you are 'metabolically negative' (you do not burn the excess calories and they are stored as more fat).

You need muscle to ensure you remain on the correct side of the see-saw, and are positively metabolically active. The only way to build muscle is to exercise. Physical activity of some sort. The good news is that the physical activity to build muscle tissue can be moderate.

If you were to walk only 10 minutes a day, this would have a pronounced effect on your muscles, aerobic capacity, and metabolic rate. Even more good news is that the positive effect of any exercise lasts for 24 hours - your body will continue to burn calories at a higher rate than normal. So, think about that as in investment: 10 minutes of exercise repays with 24 hours' worth of benefits.

Exercise releases endorphins in the body which not only make you 'feel good' but decrease your appetite. The endorphins take up receptors in the body, ensuring fewer receptors for ghrelin, the hunger hormone.

The benefits of exercise far outweigh the effort involved. The trick is to get motivated. Start off slowly, even a 5-minute walk around the block. As you get bored of that routine, stretch it to 10 minutes. Once you start seeing the positive benefits, let that be your motivation to start increasing your exercise:

- Increases deeper breathing, which improves metabolism
- Improves mood
- Increases muscle which utilizes more calories
- Decreases fat which decreases the bad hormones being released into your body
- Reduces your appetite
- Balances the emotions
- Releases feel-good neurochemicals such as endorphins
- Is good for your brain and your memory
- Offsets and delays disease of the brain such as Alzheimer's
- Improves the cardiovascular system

- Burns calories and burns fat
- Relaxes you and eases tension
- Puts you in an alpha-brainwave state which improves your sense of well-being
- Improves the ability to fall asleep, and the quality of the sleep
- Helps manage stress
- Improves your self-image, and therefore your inner confidence
- Reduces anxiety
- Offsets depression
- Prevents bone loss and osteo-type diseases
- Improves the alkaline/acidic ratio in your body
- Increases your longevity
- Generally improves your life

Why on Earth would you not want to exercise? Surely these benefits are worth 10 minutes a day?

I'll let you decide....

Chapter 11: The Importance of Sleep

Scientific research shows a link between insufficient sleep and obesity. Less sleep or poor-quality sleep leads to poor decision-making, such as choosing donuts for breakfast.

With poor quality or insufficient sleep, hormone production is badly affected.

- Your body produces more ghrelin, which makes you eat more.
- Your body produces less leptin, which is your satiety hormone making you feel full.
- Your body produces less growth hormone, which means less fat is consumed for fuel.
- These things lead to poor insulin regulation, which leads to a reduction in the management of fat and sugar storage.

Less sleep also leads to a feeling of stress and even anxiety, which leads to increased cortisol release. As discussed earlier in the book, cortisol is not a friend of weight loss and encourages weight gain. If you want to lose weight, achieve a normal 'balanced' lifestyle, and keep your weight stable, then you must have good quality (and at least seven hours per night) sleep.

Doctor-prescribed sleep medications disrupt your natural sleep which can lead to many of the above negative impacts. Natural sleep aids such as melatonin (something your body produces naturally) are recommended. The United States is one of few countries that do not require a prescription for melatonin.

Appendix

Other Self-Hypnosis Inductions

Dr. John Kappas Method

This method relies on three keywords—your physical key, emotional key, and intellectual key. Once you are in a comfortable position, let your mind drift to focusing on different parts of your body, starting with your hands.

Physical Keyword

Lie still and focus on your hands. You will begin to feel some physiological changes take place. Consider whether your hands start to feel hot, cold, tingly, numb, heavy, light, relaxed, etc.

Pick one feeling you can relate to, and try to match the word to the feeling. Examples: light, cool, relaxed, heavy, warm, cold, fluttery, tingly, etc. Concentrate on your hand(s) for approximately three to five minutes, and when you experience the feeling very strongly, say the word to yourself (e.g. relaxed). This is your **physical keyword**.

Emotional Keyword

The fact that you are now feeling or experiencing something in your body will create an emotional feeling. Spread the (physical keyword) feeling throughout your body. Concentrate on your breathing until it deepens. Become aware of your emotional feelings and now suggest various positive emotions (happiness, success, confidence, peacefulness, etc.). It must give you a sensation of well-being or elation. As you say the words, pause between them and become aware of any emotional change that you can feel. Determine which one resonates with you. This is your **emotional keyword**.

Intellectual Key

This is whichever you prefer of: 'Sleep!', 'Deep Sleep!' or 'Hypnotic Sleep!'. It might also be a power word that you prefer. Your conscious mind associates sleep with transferring control of your conscious mind to your subconscious. By association, 'Sleep!' is an instruction to transfer the conscious management of the mind over to the subconscious (into hypnosis).

Quick Kappas Method

Focus on your state of relaxation.
Have your eyes focus on an object until they become heavy.
Take deep breaths, with abdominal breathing.
Focus on the top of your head.

Repeat your **physical keyword**.

Work down your body, relaxing every part.
Countdown from five to zero.

Repeat your **emotional word**.

Do a 'staircase' (see section on self-hypnosis), counting

down from twenty to zero.
At zero—Deep Sleep! (or another choice)
Give positive suggestions to yourself.
Connect with the suggestions.
Count yourself out of hypnosis, from zero to five.
At five, 'Wide Awake!' '1,2,3,4,5...Wide Awake!'

Numerical Method

'As I relish time for myself I feel myself becoming more comfortable . . .
I feel a level of calmness and relaxation . . .
As I breathe, I begin to count . . .
One hundred—I feel deeply relaxed . . .
Ninety-nine—I feel deeply relaxed . . .
Ninety-eight—I feel deeply relaxed . . .
Eighty—I feel deeply relaxed. . .
As I count, I feel comfortable and relaxed . . .
As I count, I feel relaxed and allow myself to count quietly . . .
As I relax, I continue to count quietly in my head. . .
Seventy-nine—I feel deeply relaxed . . .
Seventy-eight—I feel deeply relaxed . . .
Sixty—I feel deeply relaxed . . .
As I count down quietly, my mind feels relaxed . . .
I feel my focus drifts from counting . . .
I feel my mind relaxed and drift . . .
Drifting towards a place, a comfortable place, a very special place where I can relax . . .
It is a safe place, a pleasant place . . .

Elevator Method

See yourself getting into an elevator which is going down. Imagine there are hundreds of buttons and hundreds of floors. Ask your subconscious which floor is required to reach self-hypnosis. Press that button. Feel your body going down with each floor. Let yourself relax, deeper with each floor. The deeper you go, the more relaxed you become. The more relaxed you become, the deeper you go. . .

When you reach the required floor, the doors open and you step out into your subconscious mind.

Ericksonian Self-Hypnosis
Sourced from: **http://www.selfhypnosistalk.com/how-to-do-erickson-handshake-induction-the-self-hypnosis-way/**

Before you initiate the process, choose a comfortable posture. Even sitting in your favorite chair will do. Make sure that you will not be disturbed during this process:

Begin with extending your hand in front of you as if you were going to shake someone's hand.

Some affirmative speech or music should be playing in the background.

You can either close your eyes or focus them on your hand.

Once you have assumed the handshake position, start

paying attention to your breathing.

Also, notice how your hand is simply hanging in midair.

Imagine various ways in which your arm might be suspended. You can imagine it to be floating in water or dangling from balloons.

You will notice that your hand is gradually becoming heavy.

Count backward from twenty and you will slowly feel that your hand is getting heavier.

Your hand can go up to touch your face, fall down on your lap or simply stay in its original place—whichever way it moves, it indicates that you have entered the trance state.

Betty Erickson Method

Sit in a comfortable chair with your feet flat on the floor.

Find a spot above eye level upon which to rest your eyes.

Soft focus and take in the whole room.

Try to keep your eyes open for a while anyway.

At some point, your eyes will naturally close. Just let it happen when it does.

Complete the sentence with observations in each of the three prime modalities (senses), Visual (sight), Auditory (sound) and Kinesthetic (feeling, touch, tactile sensations, e.g., air temperature, textures, etc.).

I am now aware that I **see**—(Repeat four times, four different visual observations)
I am now aware that I **hear**—(Repeat four times, four different auditory observations)
I am now aware that I **feel**— (Repeat four times, four different kinesthetic observations)

I am now aware that I **see**—(Repeat three times, three different visual observations)
I am now aware that I **hear**—(Repeat three times, three different auditory observations)
I am now aware that I **feel**—(Repeat three times, three different kinesthetic observations)

I am now aware that I **see**—(Repeat twice, two different visual observations)
I am now aware that I **hear**—(Repeat twice, two different auditory observations)
I am now aware that I **feel**—(Repeat twice, two different kinesthetic observations)

I am now aware that I **see**—(Repeat once only, one visual observation)
I am now aware that I **hear**—(Repeat once only, once auditory observation)
I am now aware that I **feel**—(Repeat once only, one kinesthetic observation).

At this stage, trance should be in effect.

Awakening

If you are lying in bed and your intention for self-hypnosis is to completely relax in order to get to sleep, then obviously no awakening is required. If you are sitting in a chair and performing self-hypnosis during your lunch break, and you now have to go back to work, drive a car, or operate machinery, then obviously you need to come out of self-hypnosis.

1. Tell your mind the session is over and you wish to be fully awake.
2. Count from zero to five. At five say 'Wide Awake!' '1,2,3,4,5…Wide Awake!'
3. Change your position (if sitting—stand; if lying down—sit or stand).

Blood Sugar/Glucose Sensitivity Test

Often the same diet that led to a person's diabetes is causing their overweight situation. I call this diabesity. Here is a test that may help identify glucose sensitivity.

This form is heavily subjective, but can help to pinpoint low blood sugar in the absence of an approved medical test.

KEY: If a person answers yes to ten or more of the issues, then there is a good chance of glucose insensitivity. This is not a scientific test, merely an indicator, and you should consult your doctor for recognized blood sugar tests:

#	Issue (alphabetical order)	Y/N
1	Abnormal craving for sweets	
2	Afternoon headaches	
3	Allergies/asthma/hay fever/skin rash/etc.	
4	Awaken after a few hours of sleep	
5	Breathes heavily or erratically	
6	Bleeding gums	
7	Blurred or double vision	
8	Brown spots or bronzing of skin	
9	Bruises easily (black and blue skin, takes a while to fade)	
10	'Butterflies,' stomach cramps or vaginal cramping	
11	Indecision, hesitation, 'stuck' feeling	
12	Cannot handle pressure or stress	
13	Chronic fatigue	

14	Chronic nervous exhaustion	
15	Cold hands and feet, poor circulation	
16	Convulsions	
17	Craving for a 'pick me up' in the afternoon (sweets, coffee, alcohol)	
18	Cries easily for no reason	
19	Depressed	
20	Difficulty getting started in the morning without coffee	
21	Difficulty falling asleep	
22	Dizziness	
23	Drinks x cups of coffee per day (this is subjective)	
24	Eats very often, gets hunger pains or faintness	
25	Eats when nervous	
26	Family history of diabetes or hypoglycemia	
27	Fatigue that is relieved by eating	
28	Faintness if meals are delayed	
29	Feeling of loss of control	
30	Frequent headaches	
31	Frequent yeast infections (candida)	
32	Gets 'shaky' if hungry	
33	Hallucinations	
34	Hand tremors	
35	Heart palpitations if meals missed	
36	Highly emotional or switching high and low emotions	
37	Hunger between meals	
38	Impotence	
39	Insomnia	

40	Inward trembling	
41	Irritable before meals	
42	Lacks energy	
43	Lack of sex drive	
44	Magnify insignificant events (blown out of proportion)	
45	Moods of depression or melancholy	
46	One or more sodas/colas daily	
47	Phobias or fears	
48	Poor memory or lack of concentration	
49	Reduced initiative	
50	Regular alcohol consumption	
51	Sleepy after meals	
52	Sleepy during the day	
53	Weakness or dizziness	
54	Worrier, feels insecure	
55	Symptoms appear before breakfast	
56	Symptoms disappear after breakfast	

Sources for Affirmations:

Daily affirmations are a powerful tool for improving your life. A good resource to explain how to create and how to use affirmations is:

www.freeaffirmations.org/free-positive-affirmations-ebook.

Another excellent resource is:
http://files.meetup.com/1977311/Affirmations.pdf.

Weight Loss Performance Agreement

Commitment

I _________________, am willing to lose weight, to embrace a new healthy lifestyle, to increase my self-worth, self-esteem, and confidence. By signing this document, I am committing to a contract between me, my subconscious, my friends, my family, and my hypnotherapist (which may also be me). All that separates me from my image of myself at my correct weight is a period of time.

Weight

I agree to be committed to this process of changing how I see myself and how I feel about myself. I know that I deserve to be happy and healthy. I can see myself at my goal weight of _________________lbs., and I understand that it is an unstoppable process of time. I will lose weight on a daily and weekly basis, and my goal weight will be achieved.

Emotions

I agree to let go of the fears that caused me to gain the weight. I will assess my emotions and see which of those serve me well, and which do not. I agree to discard the unwanted emotions.

Lifestyle

I do not welcome deprivation, and I understand that I do not have to deprive myself. This is not a diet; this is a lifestyle change. Through hypnosis, I will reprogram my subconscious to make better choices: better food choices, better lifestyle choices, better exercise choices. I agree to find healthier solutions for dealing with my stress. I agree to let go of a lot of things I have carried with me. This is unwanted baggage, and I give myself permission to let go.

Nutrition

I understand that when I eat 'good' foods, they act as a medicine. I understand that when I eat 'bad' foods, they have a negative effect on my body's functions and weight. I understand that looking good is a higher priority than feeding a temporary craving. A five-year-old cannot control their behavior, but I can. From this point on, I control my cravings, and my cravings do not control me.

I Am Important

I agree to make myself my number one priority. I am still committed to providing love and care for my family and others, but I realize that if I am not functioning at 100%, then I am not able to fulfill this wonderful obligation. I agree to make more time for myself, follow my bliss, be creative, laugh more and stress less. I understand that life on Earth is temporary—I might as well enjoy it while I am here!

I understand that any and all of the above contractual obligations will lead to an automatic and inevitable process of achieving my ideal weight, of ________ lbs.

I commit to:

- Stopping sabotage
- Stopping emotional eating
- Turning my body into a fat-burning machine
- Increasing fat-burning of the body (while I sleep)
- Programming myself for success and consistency
- Making my stomach shrink (Virtual Gastric Band)
- Increasing my desire to move my body
- Curbing my appetite and stabilizing my blood sugar
- Eating more slowly and mindfully
- Rejuvenating my body and supporting my health
- Eliminating my bad habits
- Programming a positive self-image
- Increasing my desire for healthy, wholesome foods
- Feeling happier, healthier and more vital
- Doing affirmations every day
- Doing ten minutes of light exercise every day, even if only walking

Signed____________________________________Dated___________
_____

About the Author

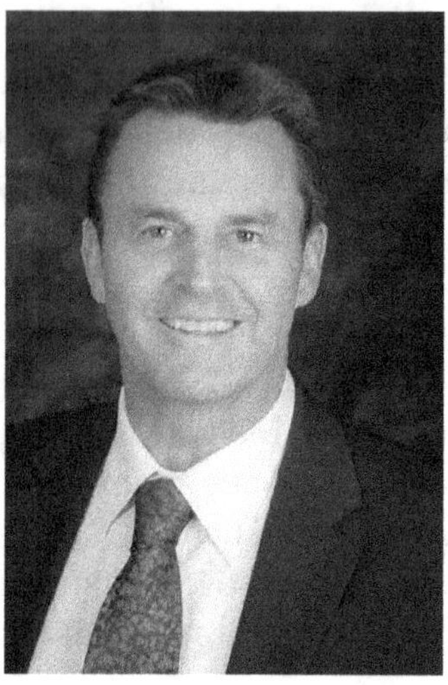

Steve Webster

An accomplished former IT and financial industry CEO, with an extensive professional background, Steve Webster decided to leave his decades-long career in the corporate world of banking and technology, to follow his passion and study hypnotherapy. He soon came to realize the incredible power of hypnosis and other modalities and began to develop programs using hypnosis to assist people in overcoming obstacles, such as weight loss. With the program and techniques he developed, Steve founded the first ever hypnosis, weight loss and wellness center in the United States: Thinessence.

Thinessence is a beautiful place in Southern California where mind and body connect to experience amazing results. Seeing in his clients that weight loss is such a personal issue that many people have struggled with for years, Steve began to feel that helping people at Thinessence was just not enough. So he decided to put his weight loss program into a comprehensive book that could reach across time zones, to help those most desperate to lose the weight. Steve's passion project became this book; with its core message: YOU have all of the tools you need WITHIN you, to achieve anything you desire, including weight loss. You are already *Thin From Within*.

Steve is a regular contributor to hypnosis media, including radio and Hypnosis TV. He is the inventor of 'Consciousness Engineering', and holds an MBA degree from Heriott-Watt University.

www.ingramcontent.com/pod-product-compliance
Lightning Source LLC
Chambersburg PA
CBHW070831260726
48654CB00025B/918